Posthuman Community Psychology

Posthuman Community Psychology is an exploration of mainstream psychology through a critical posthumanity perspective, examining psychology's place in the world and its relationship with marginalised people, with a focus on people with disabilities.

The book argues that the history of modern psychology is underpinned by reductionism and individualism, which is embedded within the contemporary psychology that we know today despite the challenges from critical and community psychologists who seek a more empowering, inclusive, and activist psychology. The posthuman community psychology ideas that emerge in this book examine and intersect with mainstream psychology, critical and community psychologies, critical posthumanities, and disability studies to propose an imaginative, reflective, and relational new psychology that represents a collection of possibilities that do not remain entrenched in older ways of thinking about humans and human connections. Richards proposes that psychology has the potential to evolve and make a powerful and profound difference for marginalised people, but a genuine desire for change from psychologists is essential for this to happen.

Illustrating the important considerations needed when examining the relationship between the discipline of psychology and marginalised people, this book is fascinating reading for community psychology students and academics, aspiring professional psychologists, community workers, and policy makers.

Michael Richards is a senior lecturer in Applied Health and Social Care, Community Psychologist, and Chartered Psychologist at Edge Hill University, UK.

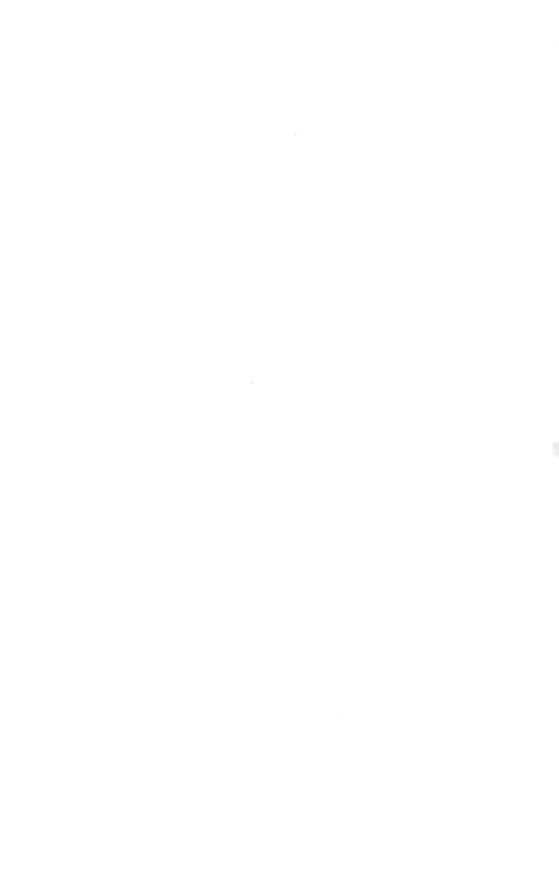

Posthuman Community Psychology

A Psychology for Marginalised People

Michael Richards

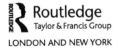

Routledge
Taylor & Francis Group

LONDON AND NEW YORK

Designed cover image: ©Getty Images

First published 2023
by Routledge
4 Park Square, Milton Park, Abingdon, Oxon OX14 4RN

and by Routledge
605 Third Avenue, New York, NY 10158

Routledge is an imprint of the Taylor & Francis Group, an informa business

© 2023 Michael Richards

British Library Cataloguing-in-Publication Data
A catalogue record for this book is available from the British Library

Library of Congress Cataloging-in-Publication Data
Names: Richards, Michael (Senior lecturer), author.
Title: Posthuman community psychology: a psychology for
marginalised people / Michael Richards.
Description: Abingdon, Oxon; New York, NY: Routledge, 2023.|
Includes bibliographical references and index. |
Summary: "Posthuman Community Psychology is an exploration of
mainstream psychology through a critical posthumanity perspective,
examining psychology's place in the world and its relationship with
marginalised people, with a focus on people with disabilities"—
Provided by publisher.
Identifiers: LCCN 2022053846 (print) | LCCN 2022053847 (ebook) |
ISBN 9780367523893 (hbk) | ISBN 9780367523886 (pbk) |
ISBN 9781003057673 (ebk)
Subjects: LCSH: Psychology. | Community psychology. |
People with disabilities—Psychology.
Classification: LCC BF121 .R447 2023 (print) |
LCC BF121 (ebook) | DDC 150—dc23/eng/20230222
LC record available at https://lccn.loc.gov/2022053846
LC ebook record available at https://lccn.loc.gov/2022053847

ISBN: 978-0-367-52389-3 (hbk)
ISBN: 978-0-367-52388-6 (pbk)
ISBN: 978-1-003-05767-3 (ebk)

DOI: 10.4324/9781003057673

Typeset in Bembo
by codeMantra

My Dad, Robin Richards
1946–2022
My son, Robin Richards
Yma o Hyd
(Still Here)

Contents

Acknowledgements

A big thank you to Dr Lucy Gibson and Dr Katie Wright-Bevans for taking their time and energy to read this book and review it for me. The positivity made me feel good and relieved after this emotional rollercoaster of writing, but the critical commentary was thought-provoking and added value to the book.

Many of the ideas, reflections, and provocations in this book are directly and indirectly influenced by the excellent scholarship and professionalism of people who I have worked with, been supervised by, or the work of people where I admire their ideas. I am sure I will continue to be provoked and awakened by their work way into the future, including the works of Professor Carolyn Kagan, Professor Rebecca Lawthom, Professor Dan Goodley, Professor Katherine Runswick-Cole, and their allies and collaborators.

A thank you to Dr Alison Moore, her collaborators, and students from the MA Social Science Critical Autism Studies programme at Edge Hill University, a programme designed and delivered with support from autistic people, for the critical discussions around some of the ideas and reflections that have emerged in this book. I would also like to thank my counselling students who have been a great source for hard debate and discussion with the ideas presented in this book.

Whilst the many marginalised groups and people I have worked with will not get a chance to read this book, their ideas, imaginations, insights, jokes, and experiences underpin the best parts of this book, and they will continue to inspire and be at the heart of my teaching and writing.

Prologue

Michael Richards

The year 2083
Silence. Shshshshshshshshshs ....
Nothing but silence. Waiting for time to move forward, waiting for answers, waiting for conclusions, wondering who I am.

I am standing in a quadrilateral room – straight, linear, narrow, and functional like a laboratory – a room that is bright white, a silver floor, all clean and mechanical, shiny, and perfect, but empty. No smells, but the smell of bleached cleanliness, with just brightness and blankness, all static and still, with no humanness.

A buzzy sound emerges in this blank and unempathetic room at the end of this white incubator. An upside-down pyramid of light appears from the floor, and a face emerges from it that is so real, but not real, with no emotion or connectivity to life. It is in the brightness that you realise that the ceiling and wall are full of circles, black circles, moving eyes, circles within circles, moving as fast as Dali's clocks (famous artist and art piece). Something is judging, labelling, and ticking boxes on a Likert scale.

The posthuman face of a Big Brother type character (a character or organisation that exercises total control) starts to speak in a monotoned but crisped voice of a Jor-El, father of Superman (character from DC Comics), who in a similar fashion had told his son what he will be:

> *Species1983 you are 38 years old. You have no gender or identity other than what I tell you what you are. I am your psychologist, and I will tell you why you are odd, unusual, weird, strange, and not of this world. You are consistently non-compliant, controlling, over-organised, vague, a poor communicator, insensitive, over-sensitive and rule bound. You hate change that is good for you. Other species say you are an idiot and other species say that you are a genius. Species say you are quiet, and species say you never shut up. Species say you are anti-social, and species say you never leave them alone. You are unloved and are loved. You are pitied, and you are hated. You have a problem with looking at eyeballs. You are a human and not of this posthuman world. My conclusion is simple. You will be labelled for life with a range of disabling labels and this will help you to conform*

to the species world around you even that you are different. You will be a part of the community of species, but always on the periphery. My judgment is complete, you may now go.

As Species1983 listens to the analysis provided by the posthuman head displayed, Species1983 feels like a psychologised, pathologised, technologised, and individualised human problem. Why exist? Why bother?

Reflections and positionalities – Who am I?

Michael Richards

Space, time, energy, data, and matter comprises what makes up the multi-verses that encompass aspects of the Marvel films that have presented imaginary beings and worlds in mainstream Western culture for years. A multiverse is the idea of different and multiple universes being in existence, which may alternate or may be parallel with our universe or different universes. This has been analysed through science fiction, physics, religion, philosophy, psychology, and literature, where debates have emerged directly or indirectly that raises questions about whether they exist or not, and therefore questions are raised about our own existence concerning what we are and what we might become. These scientific or fantastical ideas of multiverses are not what this book will be about and as the book develops, it is not going to become the next script for a Star Wars film, but the scene in the prologue could be a clip from a Marvel film or from Star Trek, a story of robots and machines, with a brief imaginative account of a character without a 'human' name. We have seen talking heads in science fiction and seen objective, monotone beings that show no emotion and empathy for the judgements being made. Usually, these films or stories depict heroes and villains, with the hero always winning, rather than witnessing any transformative change or knowing what becomes of the characters, with the hero more often or not representing the ideals of the authors and the times and contexts they live in. In the context of this prologue, the speaking head, robot, or human, who knows, is saying that for the character to survive the world they find themselves in, they must be labelled, branded, and pathologised in a way that leaves no choices. This means that the character becomes a new identity, decided by a machine or others controlling that machine.

The scene in the prologue implies that it takes place in the future, but for some readers, aspects of the scene will already feel familiar. For example, there are online doctors that make online diagnoses without physically seeing their patients or apps that can give you information that leads to self-diagnosis, some of which we saw exasperated further during the Covid-19 pandemic. However, for now, to be given a full mental health assessment in a UK context, this involves more intense scrutiny and consideration before the final label is established in face-to-face meetings. But what is likely to be familiar with many who have been involved with being assessed for their mental health, in a similar tone as the robot in the prologue, is the lack of empathy, the decontexualisation, the psychologising and individualising that people experience when being assessed or diagnosed for conditions such as Autism Spectrum Disorders (ASD). Could the prologue offer a possible futuristic outlook of how an adult could be diagnosed with ASD or is it no different than what people experience currently in mental health and medical systems?

Nobody really knows what will happen in 60 years' time, but we can certainly have a guess with the knowledge that we do have in front of us. I would suggest that the diagnosis and labelling of people with ASD or disabilities or mental health conditions will not be a lot different than today than it will be in the future as it stands, other than the fact that the process might become more technologised. Will the talking head really be a human infused in technology advancement that comes to life, when needed? Will technology think like a human because it is human made, even if it takes on a lifeform in itself? Are we already at this stage of 'human' development? These questions raise further questions on what a 'human' is and what it means to be 'human'. We only have some insights into these questions concerning technology and humankind, and who knows what might happen in the future, yet the feeling is that however technology is used to determine what diagnosis someone is given, it does seem to have similar underpinnings as medical models we come to know in physical and mental health settings in the present.

My personal insights into this are in part connected to witnessing marginalised people such as those with disabilities and mental health conditions being treated as lesser in my work as a critical community psychologist, whether in the community, working in health and social care or from within academia. In the context of this book, marginalised people are those that are treated as insignificant, peripheral or are relegated to a powerless position with a lesser voice, which includes groups and individuals I have worked that have been homeless, disabled, and experienced mental health difficulties. It was clear to me that their marginalisation within the systems I have worked in were underpinned directly and indirectly by medical models that pathologise, individualise, and psychologise people. On a personal and individual level, when I went through the process of being assessed for ASD by a psychologist, like the character in the prologue, I also felt the coldness of the person in front of me and recognised the chillness of simplified comments that were decontexualised and focused on individualised behaviour, with no assurances of what the judgements would lead to and what effects the judgements would have on the rest of my existence. Added to that was the fact that I challenged the judgements, and the more I challenged, the more the judgements became more definite and emphasised. Once you are locked into this psychologised and medicalised discourse, it aims to keep you there and whether you voice your opinions or sit in silence, the pathologising never leaves. In this instance, the psychologist decided that he wanted a second opinion, and I interpreted this decision that the psychologist wanted to label me officially, to give me a concrete, permanent label, a diagnosis of ASD, a label I would not be able to shake off if I wanted the label no longer. I felt that the label would hinder me rather than help me like I have seen with others, and so I never returned to face my 'final judgment' and I took control of the situation. Nonetheless, the process accentuated the many issues I have thought about for a long time with how society views disabilities, mental health and what 'human' is, alongside the reluctance by society to intersect humans with sexualities, genders, ethnicities, and all other factors that make us the all-round diverse people that we are. It raises questions about what being 'human' is and whether 'human' is something from a different time, and maybe 'human' is an out-of-date concept, particularly when exploring what 'psychology' means. It led me to ask further questions, and more questions after that, which would imply that the simplified way we understand labels, humans, identities, and psychology, is not viable. Some of my reflections relate to these kinds of questions:

1   To what extent are we 'human' and what is 'human' if we exclude, label, and marginalise 'Other'?
2   Does being 'disabled' inform us of what a human is or is not, and either way, should our mis-/understandings of 'disability' be at the heart of what a 'human' should be?
3   Is psychology an out-of-date discipline that reinforces disablism and promotes exclusionary practices and therefore, should psychology change to become a discipline of hope, a potential science for the people?
4   Can psychology be a force for good for marginalised people, and if so, does psychology need to be reinterpreted and redefined? What can psychology learn from other disciplines?
5   If we question our understanding of what 'human' is, does it disrupt the Western notions of ideologies such as 'person-centred care' and 'person-centredness' and whether this is the best way to help and support people if we are questioning what 'human' is and what it becomes?

To be able to start to reflect on these questions and many others, this book aims to explore the intersections through 'humanhood', 'psychology', and how this might connect with our understanding of marginalised people and in most parts of the book, relating to 'disabilities' or 'disabled people' because much of my work has been with this marginalised group. The narrative, stories, and perspectives that are shared in this book aim to challenge the deep-rooted 'certainties' of what it means to be 'human' in the context of psychology (mainstream and other psychologies such as critical/community psychology) as I have found them in my personal and professional contexts. Importantly, the book will seek to challenge the reader to rethink the idealist, narrow and unreachable notion of being a 'human' that is arguably contributes to the exclusion of marginalised people who are disabled by society.

Psychology as a discipline plays a part in that, but the book also offers hope of how we can reconsider psychology in the context of the 'posthuman', critical posthumanities, and critical/community psychology. The book, therefore, is about all people because we are all marginalised at some point, and we all call ourselves human and psychology is the study of mind and behaviour. Our understanding for what 'being human' means is multifaceted, messy, diverse, and complicated, more than ever, and thinking about this in relation to people who are marginalised or people with disabilities and in hopeful ways of what psychology can become, is a useful way to reflect on these complexities.

Guiding narrative tools – Critical autoethnography and queerying

This book is aimed at aspiring, mainstream, critical and community psychologists, as well as community workers of every kind, policy makers, academics, and students and people across different disciplines, to illustrate some reflections on what psychology means, what psychology means to marginalised groups and what it means to be 'human' at least from my perspective. The book is then a provocative and reflective exploration of those themes, with an overarching consideration of what it means to be 'human' in ever-changing political and technological times. Whilst exploring some of the big issues with psychology, the book will also seek to invoke some ideas or resolutions on how a critical posthuman perspective can help us to think differently about psychology. The ideas and reflections that emerge are informed by ideas from critical/community psychology, critical posthumanities and critical disability studies with consideration given to the idea of a 'posthuman community psychology', where psychology can be used as a stronger force for good. By doing this, the book seeks to challenge the long-aged humanist paradigm that has influenced how we think and behave as 'humans' and psychologised 'human'. This provokes reflections on whether the current discipline of psychology (in its many forms, approaches, and methods) has really moved with the pace of the ever-changing nature of what it means to be human or remained doggedly stuck within reductionist, post-positivist, and empiricist boundaries.

Whilst the book is not driven by the voices of people with disabilities or marginalised groups directly or psychologists or other professions or workers that might be relevant to the arguments posed in this book, the book will scribble down a series of reflections that draw on my work within academia, health and social care, and personal experiences, to put points in perspective. This book in essence is a critical reflection of my journey as a critical community psychologist over the past 15 years and not a demand on how people should think, behave, or change, but it might help readers to reflect on their own experiences within and on the boundaries of psychology and when working with marginalised people. To be able to do this, I will be influenced by two guiding tools, which will help me to fuse the narrative together, including critical and 'queerying' autoethnography.

Critical queer autoethnography

Holman-Jones (2016) reminds us that when using the word 'critical', it implies that knowledge is not static, permanent, or definitive, but that theorising is forever in flux, meaning that theories and ideas continue to be and need to be new, changeable, and flexible. This is important to me because as a qualitative researcher and critical community psychologist, who is not stuck on one paradigm of thinking or one discipline and is open-minded by all aspects of what psychology can offer, I look to go beyond psychology and in-between, and being intersectional allows the nuances of experience, knowledge, and perspective to emerge to provide a more well-rounded viewpoint. For me then, it becomes a better told story that encompasses the historical, social, political, and cultural aspects of our lives, but in the context of the book, specifically my own. It means that whether I directly call upon specific experiences, personal, academic, or work-related, when discussing key themes, that does not mean that this is 'it', this 'is' the way to think about the theme, because the very nature of being critical suggests that nothing stays the same, and that there is always change. This is useful for the developing narrative of this book because a critical posthumanities thread will emerge and what encompasses one aspect of this area of thinking is that we are relational and changeable beings. This is suitable when exploring 'scientific' and complicated disciplines like psychology that are arguably diverse, interpretivist and not a set discourse that sits statically ready to be prescribed to others even that aspects of psychology do just that. In other words, a critical commentary will develop with 'honest' reflections of what has directly and indirectly influenced the emerging narrative in a similar way to Parker's (2020) critical autoethnographic approach in reflecting on his journey through the teaching and practice of psychology, and Goodley (2021), who went beyond writing extensively about disability studies to writing something more personable and accessible to a non-specialist reader interested in exploring aspects of disability. Their writings have made me think that I could not possibly write this book without thinking about my own position, identities, and perspectives, and this means that to make sense of the big themes and disciplines I will explore, I will draw on my own personal stories and examples to highlight key points in the book. For example, within the chapters, there will be vignettes of professional, community work and personal experiences that will amplify some of the key points that will be made. In some chapters, I will apply some 'wonderings and wanderings' (see Morris, 2018), where I reflect and relay some imaginative visions of what could be, which adds a personable and reflexive feel to the book, helping psychology to come alive and feel ready to go beyond its perimeters of mainstream psychology, making it feel real to me as I live and be.

Whilst critical autoethnography provides the basis of a flexible and in-flux narrative, what also emerges is a reflection and analysis around identities. The book is not about specific people like it would be for a biography for instance or a life story like an autoethnography, but my identities run through the book, and this ensures that the language used will be contradictory, bias, subjective, messy, and at times confusing in the quest to amalgamate the ideas of the book together. In this respect, the use of *'queering'* helps to appreciate the fluid, playful, and political lived experiences of the workings of power and identity that circumnavigates through queer theory (Butler, 1993). 'Queerying' is not exclusively about the theorising of LGBTQIA+ identities and the book is not directly considering genders or sexualities. However, queerying autoethnography is a tool that will help me to *queery* the knowledges that oppress marginalised people such as disabled people, that is reflective in mainstream social structures and culture, and to some extent disrupt the essentialist views that come with humankind and identities that become 'norms' (also see Foucault, 1978). Indeed, the fact that this book is by default a critical commentary on the discipline of psychology and specifically mainstream psychology, it is fitting that by queering psychology and its relationship with disabled people and other marginalised groups, the book may help to 'disturb(s) the order of things' (Ahmed, 2006:161). This may challenge the relational and political orientations that stifle the identities of disabled people and other marginalised groups and thus cause a fuzziness and open up reflections on between what might be deemed 'normal', the human 'normal'. In turn, this destabilises the certain and fixed notions of identity and humanhood, which influence our understandings in our relationships and representations of others. Gibson-Graham (1999) and Slater (2015) used queerying to great effect, where they wrote with open minds and sought out the possibilities of change. In a similar way to Slater (2015), I use theory and perspectives where needed, but I am comfortable to call upon reflections of experience, personal, or professional, to make some sense of the identities and their complexities within the narration or practice, in a way that is passionate, embodied, emotional, and intellectual (Roets & Goedgeluck, 2007). Overall, the book will not be an autobiography, but a critical reflection of psychology (in its many facets) and what it is and what it can become through the lenses of critical/community psychology, critical posthumanities, and critical disability studies, without ignoring the influences of my own identities and experiences that will inevitably have some influence on my reflections.

Disabilities, marginalised people, and psychology – A messy relationship

With the book aiming to critically consider my identities, behaviours, and practices, directly and indirectly, as I write the narrative, the intellectual roots to the book have also developed and become entangled with me, so when did I first recognise the problematic relationship between disabled people/

marginalised people and psychology? In earlier publications, I recalled some of my frustrations with health and social care (Richards, 2014a; Richards, 2015a; Richards, 2016a; Richards, 2019), whether that be relating to the judgements made about the care of my family members, for example, the quick judgements made about personalities and background, or the power relations, judgements, and predictions made on people I worked with in various health and social care jobs and voluntary work. In some of these publications, I recall the prejudice, discrimination, the lack of care, and empathy that the young people and adults with disabilities received that I worked with, sometimes in blatant and at other times in subtle ways.

Those experiences at the time, and now, remind me of why I have a complicated relationship with my own discipline of psychology. For example, I feel proud to have achieved lots in the name of 'psychology', and yet, I fully recognise that psychology's individualistic standpoint and ignorance of marginalised groups in context (Kagan et al., 2021) has ensured misery and suffering for many. This leaves me in the middle somewhere from an intersectional position of seeing psychology not as a standalone subject, but a subject, a theme, a perspective that is continuously moving and becoming more diverse, and yet somehow stays the same. The individualism and scientific nature of psychology is as powerful as ever, and this is reflected in psychology's relationship with disabled people and other marginalised groups. This can be reflected in some of psychology's history, particularly relating to the understanding of 'intelligence' (see Kaufman, 1999; Stephens & Cryle, 2017), and it can also be reflected on more recent times through clinical practice and diagnosis, where the fuzziness of mental disorders and disabilities are in constant flux and misinterpretation (see Bertelli et al., 2015). In other places, I have alluded to labels being attributed to me by friends, colleagues, and psychologists. I have thought about this and how I have been labelled as 'odd', 'weird', and 'freak', amongst other words that are often used to describe people with ASD or people with intellectual disabilities (Richards, 2016b). For example, I considered the issue relating to Asperger's Disorder, which was taken away from the fifth edition of the Diagnostic and Statistical Manual of Mental Disorders (DSM-V, see American Psychiatric Association 2013), meaning that as a specific disorder, Asperger's arguably no longer exists. For me, this brought into question the strong and medicalised stranglehold that the psychiatric, medical, and health professional world has on what counts as 'disability'. In my view, the DSM was created by and is maintained by professionals from clinical and medical backgrounds, who work in laboratories, non-community/societal places, where they engage in scientific trials, ignoring the political, cultural, social, relational, and discursive consequences of disabilities. The terminology used to describe people with ASD is individualistic, talks of deficits, psychologises, and pathologises people. Essentially, these processes imply that you are brain damaged, meaning that disabilities are a medical issue and can only be resolved by science and medicine. This is something which the neurodiversity movement of the late 1990s rejected and instead attempted to push for a paradigm shift from a pathology paradigm to a neurodiverse paradigm of viewing people as different as a way of being rather than a pathology (Chapman, 2019). However, it is not helped when many charities, health care professions, policy documents, and people in power will almost exclusively use words that are medical and scientific in nature like the DSM or through medicalised and scientific discourses, even when the central ethos of their manifestos and mission statements talk about putting 'people first' and being 'person-centred'.

This contrasts with many of the ideas and perspectives that have emerged in disability studies over the past 60 years in the UK and beyond. For instance, the social model of disability helped to bring the political and social to our conversations and practices concerning disabilities (Oliver, 1990; Barnes, 1991; Shakespeare & Watson, 2002). In more recent years, the developments within 'critical' disability studies have emerged to go much further than traditional binaries of social vs. medical, to open spaces for new ideas, reflections, and interpretations that intersect with multiple identities whilst challenging the dominance of the Global North (see Meekosha & Shuttleworth, 2009; Grech, 2009; Grech & Goodley, 2012). These murmurings and challenges have helped disability studies to become more of a transdisciplinary space that opens itself up to different philosophies such as postmodernist (Shakespeare & Corker, 2002), post-structuralist (Tremain, 2005) and posthuman thinking (Goodley et al., 2016). Whilst critical realists would say that without binaries such as disabled versus non-disabled, we cannot support people properly (Vehmas & Watson, 2013), the multidisciplinary influences that have influenced new ideas and provocations in the study of disabilities have helped to dent the material dominance of social analysis of disabilities to something that is more discursive, cultural, and relational perspectives (see Shildrick, 2007, 2009; Campbell, 2008; Roets & Goodley, 2008). Could the ideas emerging in this area also be useful for psychologists and the discipline of psychology?

The development of multidisciplinary disability studies meant that thinking about disability started to go beyond just considering the political, social, and cultural aspects of disabilities to other facets that are usually ignored or lack consideration such as intimacy, sex, and sexualities (Hughes & Paterson, 2006; Liddiard, 2014; Richards, 2017). Meekosha and Shuttleworth (2009) suggested that critical disability studies are important because it builds on the multiple interdisciplinarities that encompass disability studies, including work from the global South and queer, postcolonial, indigenous, and feminist perspectives (Goodley, Liddiard & Runswick-Cole, 2017). This ensures that critical disability studies have disrupted the boundaries of humanhood, moving away from the rigidity of the holistic, ideal human, and contrasting with the principles that underpin powerful forces within mainstream psychology and humanistic psychology. Thus, when talking about what 'disabilities' means, it is very difficult to agree on one overall label because of the rhizomatic, dynamic and intersectional nature of disabilities, yet the established medical models and mainstream psychology do not view people in this way. If 'disabilities' cannot be defined, pinned down to a specific label that is permanent, fixed, and absolute, and instead, be seen as fluid and heterogeneous, then why not think about psychology in this way, which might positively affect how psychologists work with disabled people and other marginalised groups. This perspective could be useful for psychology more than ever because as Watermeyer (2012) points out, psychology is considered oppressive by supporters of the social model of disability because of psychology's ignorance of social factors that influence people with disabilities (Oliver, 1990). However, there is evidence of in-roads with psychology that are more open to different ideas that view people as dynamic and intersecting such as through aspects of community, peace, and liberal psychologies (see Blumberg, Hare & Costin, 2006). These psychologies have sought to look beyond the pathological to get a better idea of how effective psychology can be in ways that are participative and collaborative with marginalised groups (see Goodley & Lawthom, 2005a; Goodley & Lawthom, 2005b; Kagan et al., 2021). Watermeyer (2012) also proposed that instead of seeing the history of disability and psychology in terms of the 'pathological', we should go within psychology to understand psychology to get a better idea of the issues that come with this relationship, and that aspects of psychology can be an advantage for disabled people. For example, a combination of liberation and feminist psychological traditions (Martin-Baro, 1994; Lykes & Moane, 2009; Richards, 2014a) may help to understand disabilities and the social factors related to this label more, with critical engagement from within psychology rather than just dismissing it altogether. Indeed, it could be a mistake to ignore psychology because it could help to form a critical analysis to understand humanhood and disabilities better. To simply reject psychology is a problem because it will be harder to unpack the subjective and intersubjective spaces in which humans/disabilities/disabled people are forged within, and from this, we can then understand the depths oppression further (Watermeyer & Swartz, 2008). It would suggest then that to understand disabilities, an acknowledgement of societal, cultural, and political rhizomes needs to be in place and psychology can play a part in that, albeit in a revised format that dismisses its individualistic and 'royal science' ambitions (Braidotti, 2017, 2019). But, in what way can psychology develop that provides a perspective that challenges the individualistic and psychologising paradigm of psychology that has brought misery for marginalised people?

Community psychology – Hope and change?

With so many questions and concerns being raised about the relationship between psychology and disabilities, good and bad, where could I find some hope for change where psychology could be a force for good? I had already started to see hope in one specific area of psychology that I had started to engage with during my work with young people in the community as an undergraduate psychology student (Kagan et al., 2011; Lawthom et al., 2012) and could see some hallmarks on the possibilities of what psychology could become, and that was 'community psychology'. I recognised quickly that this was a psychology that was an area that did not just challenge some of my developing criticisms with psychology, but it was a discipline that offered ways to make a difference and make real change for marginalised people.

I was to find, however, that community psychology like mainstream psychology was contested in terms of what it is and what it represents because of the many different ideas that have developed in different places in the world for people who are interested in community psychology. Yet, one specific area of community psychology that was to play a major part in my development, practices and works was 'critical community psychology' (Kagan et al., 2021). This offered a framework for forming alliances, participatory work, a values-based ideology, concerned people in context and ecology, and linked in with other disciplines and professions, meaning that this psychology was not a static discipline, but one that infiltrated and fuzzed up against other ideas, perspectives, activisms, and philosophies in a way that I had never seen psychology as being. For me, values of stewardship, justice, and community (Kagan et al., 2021) became my buzzwords when working in the community over mainstream psychology's buzzwords relating to psychologising and individualising, and the ecological metaphor that links with ideas that underpin concepts such as 'communities of practice' (Wenger, 1998) all seemed the way psychology should be because it connected to marginalised people better.

I saw critical community psychology as an approach that provided hope and change within a discipline that for me had been wholly disablist, individualistic, and exclusionary from the perspective of some of the psychologists, disabled people, and other marginalised groups I worked with in the community, mostly in areas of Manchester, UK. All aspects of community psychology, mainstream or critical (discussed in more detail later in the book), arguably aim to be driven by values, working with people in context, interdisciplinary, driven by change and creative in its approaches, and can be connected to the 'humanistic psychology' that emerged in the mid-20th century, a branch of psychology that rejected much of the power force that makes up what psychology is arguably today – scientific, logical, reductionist, and reasoned. But, if one of the aims of the book is to interrogate what it means to be human in the 21st century, does the value-based approach of community psychology stand up well enough? What are the values? Who says what the values should be? What is the 'ideal' human? These questions suggest that on the surface, community psychology approaches in all their varieties, are a powerful force against the individualism of mainstream psychology. However, it could also be argued that community psychology (in whatever form) has an unstable foundation that is still essentially built upon white, middle-class, wealthy, mostly male, and Western perspectives of the 'human', which do not just underpin much of what makes up the historical and present mainstream psychology that is powerful and established but is also stuck in time compared to the futuristic and ever-changing disciplines such as disability studies, that has arguably gone through a 'posthuman' turn (Abrahams, 2017). Is it time psychology and community psychology moved with the times? If 'humans' and the world is always changing, then psychology needs to keep changing as well?

Humanistic psychology and psychology's 'crisis'

With aspects of critical/community psychology being grounded in humanistic psychology principles of the whole person, free will, the human 'condition' with self-actualising tendencies and the celebration of the uniqueness of a person, it is worth stepping back to think about what this might mean. In the 1950s and 1960s, the 'third force in psychology' emerged, 'humanistic psychology' (Bugental, 1964). This force emerged as a critique of the mechanist approaches of behaviourism and the pathologising nature of Freudian and psychodynamic psychology in understanding human behaviour. 'Humanistic psychology' emerged as a counterforce, and the works of Rogers and Maslow became enshrined in more 'client-centred' approaches. Alongside the ideas of others, such as Szasz (1961), Laing (1965, 1969), May (1969), Fromm (1973) (and many more writers that have written in this area over the decades), humanistic psychology became a powerful force that immersed itself into psycho/therapies, schools, colleges, religion, and other organisations to promote personal growth, interpersonal relationships, and ongoing development (Elkins, 2009).

Also, around this time, whilst humanistic psychology becoming a 'force', social psychology was undergoing a 'crisis' in 1970s Europe, and it is no coincidence that these forces were emerging during a time of social, political, and cultural movements and upheaval in society. Gergen's (1973) work attacked the experimental nature of social psychology and objective methods, ignoring cultural, social, and historical factors that shape our behaviour, indicating that our actions are indeed fluid and dynamic and not linear and procedural. Similarly, Harre and Second (1972) argued that people are complex, and behaviour was influenced by understanding the world around them, pointing to the work of Mead and Goffman, and ideas from Wittgenstein. Basically, the idea was that a psychologist should see how the world is interpreted by community members rather than the interpretation of an out of context psychologist. These ideas during the 'crisis' called for change in the methodological and philosophical outlook within psychology and indeed led to the development of qualitative approaches being used in psychology, which have become a central part of training and professional programmes as well as university psychology programmes. How does community psychology fit in at this point? There have been contentious perspectives on when community psychology emerged, whether earlier in the 20th century in Europe or 1960s USA (Fryer, 2008), but whatever part of history you consider, community psychology as a concept emerged as a challenge to mainstream psychology for similar reasons has the way humanistic psychology developed. There was frustration that psychologists were ignoring or not considering in their work the societal issues their clients faced, and conversations began that emphasised the need for more representation from marginalised groups within psychology with more focus on prevention than treating the individual and seeking change to systems.

Though these movements or the 'crisis' emerged in the second half of the 20th century, and both humanistic and community psychology sought to challenge mainstream psychology that still exists today in many ways, and was important in helping to promote the voices of the most marginalised, these movements were establishing a new 'foundation' in how to consider psychology. Arguably, by doing so, a new powerbase in psychology emerged that was also to become immoveable and definitive in the way mainstream psychology had become, meaning that psychology is not in flux or able to move with the changing nature of what it means to be human in the 21st century. Yes, humanistic and community psychology approaches as well as person-centred approaches aimed to 'humanise' medicine and challenge the disease-focused approach to medicine (Naldemiric et al., 2016). Yes, humanistic and community psychology/person-centred approaches considered social forces to be at the root of people's day-to-day lived experiences (Proctor et al., 2006; Sanders, 2017; Murphy & Joseph, 2019; also see Richards, 2019). Yet, this has not prevented the consistent day-to-day institutional and social abuse that disabled people and other marginalised groups still face to this very day, every day. Nor has it weakened the grip of labelling, stigma and forced treatments on marginalised people. The heart of humanism psychology revolves around holistic and congruent idealism that might have been a revelation in response to the psychologising of behaviourism and psychodynamics at the times of its inception but has not remained in step with human development and human diversities in the past, present, and future to come. For instance, our history and culture ensure that disabled people are seen as objects of pity and misfortune (Hughes, 2009, 2012), and this underpins many of the attitudes of people towards disabled people in society in the past and present, alongside other marginalised groups. You only need to read about the cases of Whorlton Hall and Winterbourne, cases of care home abuse in the UK on disabled people (Richards, 2019), along with increased hate crime, exclusionary attitudes, and practices that indicate that our society is not good at being 'person-centred' or 'humanistic' towards disabled people. Also, what has psychology or community psychology done that transforms the lives of marginalised people? This is likely to be ameliorative rather than transformative at best. Of course, not all disabled people and marginalised people are treated inhumanely, and many healthcare workers, professionals, and families care and love the people they care for profusely, but the very fact that disabled people and marginalised groups are treated as 'Other' or 'different' would indicate that disabled people, and other marginalised groups, are automatically considered to be non-human, and maybe sub-human and for that to change, they must reach an ideal that represents an 'ideal human' to survive. In this respect, it is prudent that how we view disabilities, marginalisation and humanhood needs to be challenged, and psychology has played a part in that, for the good and bad, and so rethinking what psychology is and means in the 21st century needs further dialogue for it to have a chance of becoming a psychology of hope for marginalised people.

Posthumans – Psychology moving forward

If I am arguing that marginalised people such as disabled people are essentially treated as sub-human, whether from the position of disgust or hate or pity or misfortune, then does it call into question the very meaning of what it means to be 'human'? Thinking about it at face value, we are supposed to be equals, which is enshrined in law, policy, and morality in most Western contexts at least, and indeed, humanistic psychology and community psychology would in general have the same values of equality for all. The question of what it means to be human has been asked by other scholars in recent perspectives on 'posthumanism and disability' and 'dishumanism' (Goodley et al., 2014; Goodley & Runswick-Cole, 2016). These are perspectives that question what 'human' means and challenge the individualistic notions that underpin humanism because they question the 'rationalised' individual that creates a distinction between disability and non-disability (see Frigerio et al., 2018; Richards, 2019). But what is a 'posthuman' and why could this be relevant in a conversation about mainstream psychology, and community psychology alongside thinking about marginalised groups such as those with disabilities?

The ideas of what a 'posthuman' or 'posthumanism' can be stem from different disciplines, perspectives, philosophies, art, and science fiction, amongst other influences that question and interrogate what is 'human' (see Deleuze & Guattari, 1987; Braidotti, 2006; 2013; Wilson, 2006; O'Donnell, 2011; Herbrechter, 2013; Gomel, 2014). The wide-ranging ideas from this are influenced by the ontological, epistemological, scientific, and biotechnological developments of the 20th and 21st centuries (Ferrando, 2013), such as developments like through genetic manipulation and artificial intelligence. Depending on what writers of posthumanism you read, some ideas of posthumanism are in general linked with biotechnologies that somehow lead to 'humans' becoming posthumans as people who exceed the capabilities of being a human, suggesting that what we understand to be 'human' in the present arguably no longer exists (see Bostrom, 2003a, 2003b; Hughes, 2004). Whatever way you look at the analysis of the 'human' or 'posthuman', the study of 'human' raises many questions about our mis-/understanding of what 'human' is and this has consequences on how we understand psychology and psychology's own understanding of human, mind, and behaviour.

Other forms of posthumanism can be linked to postmodernism, poststructuralism, feminist theory, and cultural studies (see Halberstam & Livingston,

1995; Badmington, 2004; Ferrando, 2013) and may go beyond the 'posts' and 'deconstruction' too by helping us to consider and make sense of our flexible and multiple identities (Braidotti, 2013) rather than rely on deconstruction and the 'posts' entirely. In this respect, we begin to recognise humans in all their diversities (also see Ferrando, 2014) and go beyond the rigidity of what 'human' means, beyond the set binaries and boundaries of human vs. non-human, binaries and boundaries being a core part and epitome of what makes up mainstream psychology, humanistic psychology, and person-centred approaches to care. By applying some of the ideas of Braidotti's posthuman perspective, it could suggest that excluded groups such as disabled people cannot be 'disabled people' or the homeless just 'homeless people' because they then become a part of a binary with non-disabled people and non-homeless. A posthuman perspective arguably would then reject these binaries because it would place humans around others, not above or in comparison, side-by-side, a rejection of humanism's 'tiered values' (Braidotti, 2013; Goodley, 2014) and residues of this can be seen in mainstream, humanistic, and community psychology, in many aspects of their own complexities. Some posthuman perspectives arguably would reject the humanistic psychology values of the whole person because we do not know what the 'person' is in the first place, or what values make up that person and the person's context, suggesting what it means to be human is too messy and too tiered into aiming for self-actualisation or uniqueness that puts us above all others. You could say then that posthumanism is concerned with 'multiple belongings' (see Deleuze & Guattari, 1987; Goodley, 2007) that are relational and work across differences. This also links with the complex subjectivities that are embodied and entrenched within our relationality with other beings and the world, rejecting psychology's individualism and rejects humanism's inflexible stance (Braidotti, 2013; Goodley, 2014) because humanism (and humanistic psychology), and I would say in its many interpretations, places emphasis on rational thought and human life above all things (see Rock et al., 2014). A critical posthumanities view would argue that a decentring view, beyond the rigid values and rational processes that come with being 'humanised' is happening and is in place because of the increasing technical, medical, economic and informatic networks that are increasingly being established in 'human' development (see Wolfe, 2010; also see Richards, 2014a).

In this respect, I would argue that mainstream psychology and in certain respects, critical/community psychology, needs a rethink about its identities and a reflection on what they are in the context of ever-changing people and contexts. Psychologists need to think about what the study of mind and behaviour really means and go beyond established values of humanhood and person-centredness and focus on the relational, changing, diverse identities, and contexts that we really experience and that are influenced by wider social, cultural, political, biological, and technological aspects of life. For all humanistic psychology and critical/community psychology's determination to act and make a difference, nothing transformative or revolutionary has arguably taken place other than when the process, project, caring role, or task is ameliorative in nature, and the evidence can be seen in the experiences of the marginalised people I have worked with, and so many of which are as marginalised as ever. A rethink on how we view psychology, the 'human', and marginalised groups such as those with disabilities within a posthuman context might provide a fresher feel to how psychologists and health and social care professionals understand the people they work with. Maybe the actions, ideas, works, and behaviours of marginalised people might help us to be more effective in bringing positive change, with positive, relational, and realistic relationships with people who are experts in exclusionary practices and the permanent effects of marginalisation on their lives. A process of de-ideologisation in psychology needs to take place to enable living beings to be treated fairly as equals, as people alongside people and all living things, and this could be viewed through a 'posthuman community psychology' lens, which will be explored later in the book. In that chapter, I will present some ideas underpinned by a critical posthumanities outlook, that will act as a guide to reflect on how some of these ideas could look for psychology.

Historical, political, societal, and personal contexts

In line with the social, cultural, and political influences that are very much a part of thinking about what 'human' means and thinking about marginalised groups and psychology's roles in all this, it seems sensible to contextualise some of the historical, political, societal, and personal circumstances that directly and indirectly influence the narrative of this book. This connects back to the critical queerying of my identities, positionalities, and practice that will emerge through the book. For example, I was born in 1983 in the UK, not long after Margaret Thatcher won her second General Election in the UK (first female prime minister of the UK), and one that was a landslide victory ensuring that a Conservative political agenda would prevail for years. The Labour leader (the Opposition) was Michael Foot, who was to be compared nearly 40 years later with Jeremy Corbyn, the Labour leader from 2015 to 2020. Both Foot and Corbyn were left-wing politicians, who wanted to take politics and Labour back to the left. Corbyn wanted to move away from the ideals of New Labour (globalised capitalism and a midway point between neoliberalism and social justice, amongst other ideals) set out by Tony Blair and Gordon Brown in the 1990s (Labour prime ministers in the UK 1997–2010) whilst I was in secondary school. However, both Foot and Corbyn failed in the 1983 and 2019 General Elections, with the Conservatives winning those Elections convincingly. Furthermore, in the lead up to writing this book, the 2019 General Election in the UK had just taken place, dominated by a Brexit narrative. 'Brexit' concerned the UK leaving the European Union (EU), an organisation that is a group of 28 European countries that are politically and economically tied together, allowing for free movement across borders and the establishment of the currency, the Euro (19 countries in the EU, but not the UK), alongside other important factors including trade and environmental policy. In 2016, the people of the UK narrowly voted to leave the EU, and this led to constant division and debate for the next 3.5 years. The UK General Election in 2019 led to a Conservative majority in the Houses of Parliament, UK and a guarantee that the UK would leave the EU. This ensured that the Conservative party would likely be in power until 2025, and unless the opposition have a landslide victory, there is a possibility that the Conservative party will be in power for another 5–10 years, culminating over the same period of time as did the Thatcher-Major Conservative governments of the 1980s and 1990s. A period of time that is parallel with the present in 2022, with society facing high taxes and energy bills, recession and involved with wars in different places in the world.

As the General Election ended in 2019, the first cases of Covid-19 were emerging in China. At that point, nobody could have imagined the pandemic that was to quickly emerge across the globe and led to unprecedented controls over movement, travel, money, cultural activities, and simply day-to-day life from a walk in the park, to not even being allowed near your loved ones in your own home. One of the first key decisions and actions by the UK government, which was to directly affect disabled people and other marginalised groups, was the establishment of the Coronavirus Act 2020. The Act aimed to reorganise health and social care to align itself with the unprecedented and changing circumstances of the pandemic, but this was problematic from the start. The Act arguably suspended disabled people's rights to social care to an extent. For example, it was posited that the local authorities only needed to provide care if they considered it necessary, so choices could be made about who received care or not. This inevitably led to people suffering and likely led to death in some cases, deaths that could have been avoided. Disabled people were one of the most vulnerable groups, for many reasons, in catching this virus, and were less likely to recover than most because of underlying conditions. Additionally, the new, and hastily put together, National Institute for Health and Care Excellent (NICE) guidelines announced at the time (March 2020) that people admitted to hospital would be assessed on how frail they were. This was done using the Clinical Frailty Scale, which was created for people with dementia, not other marginalised groups. The scale has nine levels from the very fit to the terminally ill. The problem with this scale is that it did not allow judgment to be made about the intersubjective experiences of disabled people on a day-to-day basis, and alongside issues with communication and disabled people and health professionals, which is notoriously poor based on the accounts of disabled people I have worked with, there was no consultation, and this was a real cause for concern when making judgements about who should receive care or not (see Liddiard, 2020; Goodley et al., 2022). How can you place someone with intellectual disabilities on this scale? How severe or not is an intellectual disability? By using this scale, in a pressurised hospital environment, how can you really decide who has the right to critical care or not? Also, what is sometimes not acknowledged enough are the less obvious circumstances of Covid-19 that have led to social isolation and physical isolation, ensuring that people were lonely, had less accessibility in using technology, less care, a lack of money, friends, and family (see Saltzman, Hansel & Bordnick, 2020). Arguably, these questions once again suggested that in times of crisis and governmental decision-making, disabled people and other marginalised groups were not a priority, not as equal as other people. This ableism is as strong as ever in human society. Even in a global crisis, there was an opportunity to change course in attitude and to take action like never before to make the world a better place, but again, disabled people were not considered equals despite the Health Secretary of the time in the UK saying that 'we are all humans... that's what brings us together'. This once in a lifetime event in terms of its scale and influences across all groups of people and nations, was an opportunity to do something greater than ever for disabled and marginalised people, and once again when there is an opportunity for real transformative change, it did not happen, and arguably things only got worse for the most marginalised.

With the issues relating to Thatcherism in the 1980s and the issues relating to austerity in the 2010s as a consequence of the Global Financial Crisis (2007–2008) such as increased poverty, increased health inequalities, more hate crime and increased marginalisation for already excluded groups, amongst other issues (see Scott-Samuel et al., 2014; O'Hara, 2015), and with the likely recessions to come whilst Covid-19 continues, it feels like I have lived through similar political landscapes as a child and adult, a feeling of going around in circles, history always repeating itself. What is for sure, whatever way you look at it, whether it be in the 1980s or 2020s, marginalised groups are excluded within society more than ever, despite the developments in technology, science, education, medicine, and globalisation and I have seen this personally, professionally, in my research and teaching. My recollections of the late 1980s and 1990s always seem to go back to seeing bad news on the big brown televisions many people had or shocking headlines in newspapers, and I recall thinking to myself that we do not seem to live in a nice world. It is no doubt that my sense of injustice grew during these times. However, other influences during those times influenced me to, directly or indirectly, including my complex and unusual upbringing, poor schooling, the confusing and controlling aspects of Roman Catholicism at home and school, which meant certain beliefs had to be upheld, often in opposition to teenage desires and contradictions of the adults, nuns, priests, and teachers around you. Mix this in with alcoholic and drug abusing relatives, who ruled with the hand and objects, mixed in with emotional and neglectful abuse and other abuses, contradicting the demands put on me and my siblings to be god-fearing Christians, ensured that the sense of injustice, personal and beyond, was likely to prevail at some point.

I struggled in school, not academically, but with trying to be a 'good boy' whilst putting on a guise of life is normal at home, trying to live up to expectations set out by schools and family, and trying to be a normal teenager wanting to have girlfriends and have fun with friends. My frustration with life and the world around me was disabling and caused great sadness. There was always this expectation that if I did not meet the standard of my great uncle, a graduate of the University of Oxford, and a Roman Catholic priest, then you were not up to much, and that was coming from people who did not achieve much themselves. It is no wonder that I had difficulties in responding to people in power, usually domineering and ruthless characters, and expectations set out in the education system, a system that clearly suits some people over others. It was a great relief to me that before I completed my GCSE's (a qualification in the UK that children must undertake before leaving school), not long after I turned 16, that I walked out of school. I had enough of being judged, ignored, and was not able to be happy or be myself. The school and its professional associates failed to care for me and help me, like it did with many of my peers, many of whom still face great challenges in their lives, which could have been prevented in the early parts of their schooling. Everyone thought I was silly for doing it, and yes, the pressure from everyone was hard, and even more so when you are just one voice, young and vulnerable, it was a very lonely time, but I was able to start college and start again, on my terms, and redevelop my love for learning and education, not the enforcement of it by society and abusive individuals. I prospered and I was introduced to new ideas that sunk the Roman Catholicism ideologies and catechisms that I had etched in my brain, particularly when I was introduced to Marx. I really knew what Marx meant about religion being the 'opium of the people', at least from my personal perspective, that it was a powerful force that convinced you that you were always wrong. It made you feel that you could not be yourself, and this never really made sense to me considering the wide range of bad characters that had surrounded me through my life, who were preaching hypocritical, religious vitriol.

One of the other senses of injustice that I experienced growing up was the discriminatory behaviour towards my dad. My dad being a former Welsh miner from South Wales, who left Wales for England in the 1960s to find work, like many people had to do to survive and experience a better life. Yet, he faced consistent discrimination and I have many memories of hearing drunken rages from family members towards my father, using derogatory anti-Welsh language, and neighbours and gangs causing damage to the house and making threats, always with a Welsh twist to it. I remember looking on with worry and fear, looking forward to the day that I could be older to stop this from happening. I remember hearing racist, homophobic, transphobic, and anti-class vitriol throughout my childhood, in school, at home, and when I played on the streets, aimed at specific people, who just appeared to be different. Indeed, being the oldest of five children, in a two-up, two-down house added to my sense of injustice because early on I was expected to look after the children because one parent was recovering in bed for most of the day from daily cider binges, whilst the other parent would be away working. Like so many people I have worked with in the community and with students, I know what it is like to spend a whole childhood in damp conditions, always cold, a constant empty fridge and like some, if naughty or perceived to be naughty, I know what it is like to be beaten by a stick or a slipper by family members or if not 'caught', on one occasion at least, one family member picked up dog shit and threw it at my head where it remained matted in my hair for days. With my expertise now in health and social care, it is incredible that we were not taken into care, and so maybe it was not just family members that let us down. Health and social care professionals and systems that were in place that were meant to care for children and vulnerable people, let us down. Even when they visited home or raised questions at school, no action was ever taken, and looking back, it just came across as professionals not being bothered or doing their job properly and efficiently. They must have known that things were not right when they visited and did nothing, but you do not know how to make sense of it or understand any of it when you are a child – you are totally disempowered, regardless of what policy and laws are in place to promote children's voices. It raises questions about why certain choices were made in my household, such as why buy alcohol before the buying of food for starving, cold children. Why was it always cold and damp and why did I have to live a life that felt like I lived in Victorian times? There was no shower, no central heating, and always feeling unclean, with nobody wanting to be your friend or invite you to parties, the abuses always needing to be covered as a priority. I wonder if there had been social media and the Internet at the time, maybe I could have found some answers, but then again, would any of that had been affordable and would any of it made a real difference? I will never know now.

What is for sure is that despite the abusive childhood that I have endured, my sense of injustice and my sense of identity became stronger, and these influences will almost certainly influence me now and the narrative of this book, in subtle and less subtle ways. I was able to free myself of the shackles of abuse of my youth and start to think about life in a different way, and this came with my work and university life that were to add extra layers of my sense of injustice, and indeed, how I could develop into someone who could be useful, but at times could be a barrier and cause problems as well. When I first started to work in social care and volunteering organisations (for example, with young homeless people, people who had been abused or people with mental illnesses), having been influenced by the powerful and engaging works of Kagan et al. (2021) where my interests in critical community psychology emerged, I thought I could change the world. After all, I emerged from my own controlling contexts of my youth, why could I not help others and make a difference in the world, maybe even be a hero and feel good that I have done good. However, I gradually found that the organisations and the leaders who I had encountered, who enshrined themselves as leaders that were all about inclusivity, empowerment, and participation, always ready with a 'bottom-up' approach rhetoric, were in fact politicians with neoliberal ambitions, lovely people on the surface, but challenge them, and there would be nastiness. Change was key for me as a critical community psychologist, and change was key for these organisations, but change meant relinquishing power, undermining people in powerful positions, disrupting the status quo and I learned the hard way, that change was not going to happen, certainly not in a way that would be transformative. The complex power structures alongside the complicated lives and contexts of the marginalised groups I worked with made for a very messy system that prided itself on being 'person-centred', but the evidence of which was very complicated. I often say how much I miss being with those groups of marginalised people, because we also had fun, worked hard and really tried to make a difference, and I had insight and empathy of my own circumstances that made me feel connected to them. But I do not miss the disempowering and hypocritical systems that we had to work within, and I acknowledge that I am sure I was disempowering, hypocritical, and could have been more diplomatic at times as well.

In the years leading up to this, I had been a student in the psychology department at Manchester Metropolitan University, UK, and I could see what I had learnt come alive in the community through the teachings of critical psychologists, community psychologists, and disability studies thinkers. Yet, being in that department has turned out to be another 'odd' element to my experiences and development because it was like no other psychology department I have known since. The psychology department was famed for writing 'Qualitative Methods in Psychology' (Banister et al., 1994) and the department was an international centre for critical psychology and community psychology for many years. When I speak to former students now from the 1990s and 2000s, they say the same, that we recognise the powerful effects of seeing psychology differently and that psychology needed to be seen differently and that is what we gained from being in this department. We recognised that psychology could be empowering, inclusive, creative, and be a discipline that could change the lives of people and the world for the better. That being said, things changed especially in recent years, and it is maybe a sign of the times that whilst qualitative methods and aspects of community and critical psychology have emerged in accredited psychology programmes in the UK and beyond within the past 40–50 years, they were and still are essentially seen as secondary and less important and arguably fading away in some instances. For me and others, this was what psychology was and needed to be and needs to be now even that critical/community psychology and disability studies can at times be, in my experience, counterproductive and not be as transformative, empowering, participative at all levels and inclusive as they claim.

The contradictions of growing up in the metaphorical 'gutter' in my first 20 years to the more recent 20 years of success also need to be acknowledged. I have faced difficulties growing up, like so many people do, but through hard work, and at times pure good luck, I have been able to achieve and experience many things including being able to travel to different countries, achieved degrees, and have a home that I own. The greatest happiness alongside this is being a father and watching my son turn into the character that he wants to be and experience many great activities and experiences that many of us could only dream about growing up. The queerying of myself highlights that my identities are always in flux, are fuzzy, colourful, different at different times and contexts, and yet, very much in the moment it is fair to say I am a privileged, heterosexual, white, middle-class, educated man, who can own a home and develop a useful pension. This makes for a book that is hypocritical in its stance in critiquing a discipline like psychology that epitomises that identity in many ways, but it is also an acknowledgement that I am prepared to challenge myself and my position and that it should not be an all-empowering permanent fixture that dictates what is right or wrong or what is truth or not. As I will explore further in the book, I also reflect on the fact that sometimes autoethnographies or a queerying type narrative can produce an 'heroic' discourse of someone who has 'suffered' and now 'risen like a phoenix', and this discourse can be misleading because narratives cannot cover everything and every possible context and interpretation. I will concede then, that I can be a fool, selfish, ignorant, narrow-minded, and annoying, even if I do not realise it in those moments with people and this will be queeried in some of my vignettes within the book. I do not seek to be a victim or a hero or anything like that, there are some who say I am these labels and there are others who would strongly dismiss these labels. Yet, how could I not say how I feel and contextualise myself to some extent when discussing what the study of the mind and behaviour and what the human is and can be? I could not possibly position myself as a positivist, trying to be objective and reductionist, or write in that way with this book because I would not be able to consider the issues that are central to the book without doing so.

Summary of reflections

I began this introduction to the book by presenting a futuristic and technological outlook of how someone might be diagnosed with ASD in the future. I alluded to the clinical, objective, and labelling voice of the 'judge' that was not just one for the future, but that pathologising and psychologising voice has been present for a long time for disabled people and other marginalised groups and likely to continue. I linked this with my own personal experiences and presented the reasons why this book, directly or indirectly, will be a critical autoethnography that queeries the big themes and issues that are central to the book, indicating my position within it. I also briefly mentioned that the history of psychology and its relationship with disabled people and other marginalised people is problematic, but to start to develop a book that actually wants to bring some hope rather than just plain, obvious critical analysis and blasting psychology out of the water, I also referred to critical/community psychology that aims to be value-driven, contextual, and empowering for people rather than looking to fix and provide simplified outcomes to complicated difficulties. Yet, for all critical/community psychology's drive to empower and promote social justice, it is arguably enshrined in human-istic psychology's traditions of reaching self-actualisation and for people to become an 'ideal' human in a way that is not parallel with how people view the world today. In this respect, a critical posthuman perspective could offer a way for critical/community psychology and psychology to develop itself into a psychology that is fit for purpose that is amalgamated into the relational, diverse, and interconnected people that we are today, more than ever, and this will be explored further later in the book. To help put some of that into perspective, as I am one author with one narrative in this book, a brief out-line of my own background was acknowledged (at least my interpretation of it) alongside some of the political, social, and cultural influences of the past 40 years that are likely to have an influence on this book.

Some will say that too much is being considered, meaning that the narra-tive is likely to be vague, loose, hypocritical, and contradictory (much like psychology?). I understand that, but as a psychologist, where the study of 'human' behaviour is at the heart of it, it is useful to be able to try to turn that upside down and think about it in the context of disabilities and other marginalised people. By doing so, alongside reflecting on what it means to be human and to bring some hope that psychology can be a psychology for the people, whatever those people are, then it acknowledges that these themes are complicated, and psychology is also complicated. However, it could be use-ful, and I hope engaging enough for psychologists and other professionals to think harder about making a psychology a psychology of hope and a genuine force for good for all as we move deeper into the 21st century. With that in mind, I think about Braidotti's useful reflection and try to be the same with a reflective and open mind:

> Those who go through life under the sign of the desire for change need accelerations... need to be visionary, prophetic, and upbeat.
> (Braidotti, 2010: 216 – also see Kumm et al., 2019)

Mapping the book

The introduction to the book presented some of the theoretical underpin-nings and some reflections on my position and the accelerators that inspired the ideas within the book. To start to explore some of these ideas in more detail, Chapter 1 will critically examine some of the main perspectives that are underpinned by critical posthumanities to help establish the critical nar-rative of what it means to be human and how this relates later in the book to psychology, community psychology, and marginalised people. Chapter 2 will provide a brief history and one person's perspective of modern psychology, exploring psychology's foundation and structure to reflect on what contem-porary psychology looks like in the 21st century. Chapter 3 will explore a specific branch of psychology, 'critical/community psychology', to present ideas relating to social justice, empowerment, and inclusion, with some critical commentary on how far it has come, or not, in making changes and differences in psychology and beyond. Chapter 4 will explore critical/community psychology in more detail and critically reflect on why it works but does not work at the same time by reflecting on some of my professional and personal experiences whilst 'doing' critical/community psychology. Chapter 5 will present some ideas and reflections on what a 'posthuman community psychology' could be and what it could do for psychology and will present some reflections on what a new, becoming psychology could look like, with a view to refashioning the mainstream psychology that is powerful and established. Chapter 6 will end the book with some critical commentary on what a posthuman community psychology could look like in the context of disabilities and disabled people.

1 Critical posthumanities – A becoming world

To be Welsh or not to be Welsh

From time to time, I recall the many moments in my childhood where I would watch and listen to people abusing and discriminating against my dad, whether that be on my street or in our home, for being a Welsh person. I would listen to the insults like 'Welsh bastard', 'sheep shagger' (in reference to the number of sheep that live in Wales), and 'you Paki' (a racist term used against people from Pakistan, with a view to marginalise my dad in the way they did to others). Sometimes these insults were accompanied by weapons used in a threatening way. I recall when the football teams, Wrexham, or Swansea (football teams in Wales) came to Stockport (a town near Manchester, UK) to play football, our home became a target of abuse, or when Wales would play England in an international football game, in one instance, a bouquet of daffodils (a national symbol of Wales) was thrown outside the house. Bear in mind that there were no obvious indicators that the house and family were Welsh, other than hearing my dad's accent and 'knowing' that he was a Welsh person. I think when you are child and seeing this, two things can happen. First, you can be scared and be full of fear and anxieties that make you want it all to go away, seeing your beloved dad be abused in this callous way, and no doubt that is what I would have felt as a child. Or, second, you take the anger and sadness of what you witness and fight back and do not let the bullies win.

My fighting back began very early in life then, and it has not stopped. I am known for my pride in my Welsh background, and I make sure everybody knows it, whether it is when I recall my memories of being in Wales or recite stories from watching the rugby union (Welsh national sport) or boast that my dad was a miner in 'Big Pit', a coal mine and a world heritage site in Blaenavon, South Wales. Sometimes this leads to comments like, 'you are not really Welsh', 'you weren't born there',

DOI: 10.4324/9781003057673-1

'you do not speak Welsh or sound Welsh'. Accordingly, from spending a childhood watching anti-Welsh sentiment against my dad, including from within my own non-Welsh/Irish family, I am 'not Welsh' because I do not tick unaffirmed criteria that would make me 'Welsh' that relates to biology, birth and sounds of a voice. Similarly, in a way not so different, I visit Wales, and I say I am Welsh, and I am rejected there as well: The 'English cousin' rather than our 'Welsh relatives in England'. And then if I say I am Welsh to some people in northern parts of Wales, I am Welsh because it is an opportunity to mock the South Welsh people for being more 'English'. To add another dimension, I have taken a DNA test to explore my biological descent through the ages, and it confirms that I am not English, but Welsh (52%), Irish (43%), and Scottish (5%), maybe making me the ultimate, biological Celt or at least mostly Welsh; then again, there were never countries as we know them now all those thousands of years ago, making me a cocktail of all sorts of identities and possibilities.

    As a result of all this, amongst some of my experiences I referred to in my history in the introduction chapter, it is no wonder that I have been interpreted as odd, strange, Welsh one minute, when someone feels the need to insult me, English the next minute, when someone wants to insult me the other way around, and people knowingly do this, sometimes in banter, other times to be nasty, and other times to make a political point. Do I promote my Welsh identity as staunchly as I do because I am stubbornly still fighting back on my dad's behalf against the anti-Welsh sentiment of my youth or is this my identity that people choose not to accept because I do not tick their criteria for 'Welshness'? It raises the question for me, and it seems for others, 'who is Michael'?

Throughout my life so far, the rejection of my identity and witnessing my dad being marginalised for his identity because of where he was born, his accent or label of being 'Welsh' has made life complicated at times. The very essence of this means you question who you are and everything else more to make sense of it, in line with some of my personal reflections in my introduction about growing up and developing as an adult. All this, alongside the discrimination, underpinning colonial ideals, violence, aggression, and the subtle, nuanced, indirect controlling dimensions of rejection for who you are or who you feel to be over times and contexts, made me inadvertently question what it means to be human, in all its complexities, and this I will directly and indirectly continue to question and queery through the book.

    Academically, I have only recently thought directly about what it means to be human, but actually I have always questioned what it means to be human because at times I have not been treated as 'human' or I have witnessed specific groups of people being treated as 'non-human' and I am sure most people have felt this way at some point in their lives. Therefore, I have always been surrounded by question marks over what 'human' is and it is through the difficult moments you think about this more. Whilst I have experienced difficult moments, I am open-minded and realistic enough to know that many more people have faced greater difficulties than me. I noted in my introduction chapter that I am now in a privileged position, and that it was not always like that, so what have I become? It is easy in some ways to say who I am, and in other ways, it is not so easy. Many people do not get to this privileged position, because of the stereotypes, discriminations, and the labelling they face, in effect, some people will be treated as second-rate, sub-human, or the 'Others'. The reflection about my 'Welshness' has lived within me, around me, in my feelings, my identities, and my words for a lifetime, and no doubt, this will be forever. It raises questions about what it means to be 'me' and helps me to think about what 'we' might understand to be 'human' and what that has become and can become again, beyond text-book stereotypes of what you 'should be'.

I have presented a sombre tone to the beginning of this chapter; however, the chapter goes onto to present an inquisitive and queerying tone that might provide some positivity about what humans have 'become' and are 'becoming'. With the negative experiences, I have also had the great experiences, and I recognise that this is all about 'me' when reflecting on myself, but to start to think about a 'posthuman community psychology' later in this book, how can I not think about who I am and where this narrative might lead, or start to think about what it means to be 'human' in my own context? I recall Richardson and St Pierre (2005:967) when they say, 'writing is thinking... writing is indeed a seductive and tangled method of discovery', and Adams and Holman-Jones (2011:110) point out that within autoethnography, identity, and experience are 'uncertain, fluid, open to interpretation, and able to be revised'. These thoughts seem to be relevant to me as I queery my position within and outside of psychology and how I think about humanhood and change because I am always changing, and in other ways stay the same, and so does the world. To help to start to think about some of these reflections and ideas, this chapter will explore some of the ideas that encompass 'posthumanism' or the 'posthuman', and about how this is relevant to our understanding of 'human life', in the past, present, and possible future. This critical overview will infiltrate my analyses to come when exploring psychology, humanistic and critical/community psychology, and disabilities. In this way, it will help to make some sense of the rhizomatic nature of what it means to be 'human', to be me, and how it might contribute to our understanding of 'becoming'.

Posthumanisms – A brief overview

My introduction to 'posthumanism' began during the final stages of my PhD. The PhD focused on working with a group of men with intellectual disabilities, with the aim to challenge misconceptions about disabilities using visual and creative methods (Richards et al., 2018). By using community-based arts, the voices of the men were promoted with a view to challenge the stereotypes and stigma that they faced in life, alongside other marginalised groups. Alongside the development of this project, I wrote a series of autoethnographies, examining my position, emotions, observations, and contexts that influenced the research and development of the work. The autoethnographies helped me, at least to some extent, to think about who I was and who my participants were, and how our identities and contexts were similar such as through our difficult childhoods, our complicated relationships with institutions and discrimination. These reflections also indicated that despite the similarities, my role and positions, and the roles and positions of my fellow 'non-disabled' facilitators, ensured that we had roles that were powerful such as 'researcher', 'psychologist', 'student', 'facilitator' over their roles as being 'participant', observed', 'Other', and 'disabled' (see Richards, 2015a), which indicated clear binaries between us. These binaries ensured that participation, power, expertise, and inclusion were limited for some over others, and this raised questions for me about why these binaries are in place and what it means to be human. These reflections were reinforced at the time, and thereafter, through the works of Goodley and Braidotti, and their work shed further light for me on what being 'human' or a 'posthuman' means and how we view ourselves and the world (see Braidotti, 2013; Goodley, 2014, 2021; Goodley et al., 2014, 2019, 2020).

What really struck me about the 'posthuman' or 'posthumanism' (albeit varied and interpreted in many ways) was that it encompassed a range of contemporary theoretical positions from different inter/intra disciplinary backgrounds such as philosophy, literary studies, critical theory, and the arts, with some of this thinking emerging in other fields such as disability studies (Goodley et al., 2019). This was a refreshing outlook for someone who had been caged within the boundaries of mainstream psychology because despite the many interpretations of posthumanism, it is essentially concerned with breaking away from established assumptions about what 'we' are from a Western cultural perspective. Instead, posthumanism was something that felt newer and a more meaningful way to understand the 'human' and its relationship with nature and all things, and this helped me see psychology in new ways. Yes, Miah (2007) implied that the history of posthumanism is a series of disagreements about the value of being 'human' and an exploration into the social conditions for self-modification through technology has become a necessary part of human life, influenced by current socio-cultural-political processes, meaning we could around in circles, and in and out of them, trying to define 'human' and not get anyway because it is all so complicated. But Miah's (2007) point is important and relatively straightforward to understand too in the context that it indicates that humans have changed and keep changing. So, it is not a surprise that the near 50-year history of posthumanism is complex and muddled, because humans are complex and muddled and this resonated with me in my work with disabled people and my own identities. For me, this fluidity and spectrum of trying to understand what a 'human' is went some way in opening my mind up about our identities and place on earth and beyond, steering away from the established, set-in-stone values that underpin humanism. This was something that made a lot of sense to me in understanding myself and people with disabilities alongside other marginalised groups rather than be overpowered by the indoctrinating entrenchment of medicalised and psychologised perceptions of disabilities and excluded people. The kind of views for some have become norms that generally remain static and unmoveable, but often enshrined with 'humanistic' values and principles that might not fully reflect the changing nature of humans and the world around them.

My initial readings of posthumanism led me to its roots and the questions that have been asked through posthumanism in recent decades relating to what being human means. For example, Hassan (1977) is usually credited with being one of the first to use the word 'posthumanism' in his seminal work, 'Prometheus as Performer: Toward a Posthumanist Culture'. For Hassan, the humanistic dualisms of subject vs. object or science vs. culture were no longer in place. Instead, traditional distinctions were blurring, ambiguous, and diverse, which can be seen in the blurring's between science and art, and the image of 'man' and the concept of human through the developments of artificial intelligence, space travel, and organ transplants in recent decades. This made sense to me because I too could see the blurring and diversity within my work with marginalised people and my own identities in life so far, and yet, the binaries between disabled versus non-disabled or the excluded vs. included were clearly in place and made a difference in how each grouping would be treated.

Hassan and other writers of posthumanism of the time, in general, started to put forward a new idea about humanity that goes beyond Cartesian dualism and anthropocentrism (human-centred point of view of the world and ultimate moral standing over all things) to something that challenged the established boundaries and categories between living things and technology. This suggested that maybe more than ever that the line between human and non-humans and between humans is continuously changing and therefore, the anthropocentric outlook was being challenged. Indeed, the very word 'posthuman' seeks to undermine, interrogate, and reject the entrenched philosophies of Western humanism that is central to the decision-making, attitudes, politics, and day-to-day life of many people. 'Humanism', depending on where you want to start (from the philosophers in Rome and Greece to the Renaissance to the Enlightenment to Rogers in the 20th century), is anthropocentric, a historical phenomenon that has been reinterpreted time and time again in placing 'man' at the centre as opposed to God or anything or something else (see Bolter, 2016). This was understood in modern science and Cartesian terms as being able to understand the world around through reason and observation and 'man' could examine the world around them in a detached and objective way, in ways we may experience during medical

consultations or how robotics is presented to us. And, whilst the philosophical strongholds of Marxism, Darwinism, and Freudianism started to break
away from those entrenched scientific positions to some extent, the developments that grew in the 1800s into the 1900s in the fields of psychology and
biology, the positivist dichotomy of the subject vs. object, maintained itself
and can still be seen despite developments and changes in aspects of science
and psychology well into the 21st century (Bolter, 2016).

The World Wars of the first part of the 20th century made people think
differently and can be seen in modern art, politics, medical and technological developments. The postmodernists and poststructuralists also emerged
and through their deconstructions of established truths, and they were essentially laying the path for the deeper critical analysis of what the 'human'
is or became later in the 20th century. For writers such as Derrida (1997),
Foucault (1964, 1972, 1977), and Barthes (1957), they questioned the established truths and universal, Western epistemologies with critiques of language,
cultures, and political structures. Both postmodernism and poststructuralism (and some of the other posts) were critical reactions to an empire-
feeling world that exemplified the modern era that demanded universality
and simplicity. It was by the second half of the 20th century, the 'posts'
started to take shape and disrupt, in some ways, those established orders that
had cemented themselves in Western thought and application in the sciences.
The postmodernist and poststructuralist sought to challenge 'modern truths',
and by doing so, critiqued our standing in the world and beyond and this lay
the catalysts for the development of posthumanism later. Moreover, Lyotard
(1979/1984) critiqued the 'master or grand narratives' manifested within our
current ideologies within societies whether that be Marxism, institutional
religions or universal reason, ideologies that dictate an interpretation of history or how people should live. For example, Lyotard advocated for 'local'
narratives grounded in the diversity of human experience where varieties
of theoretical positions exist rather than one grand narratives. These ideas
along with poststructuralism and postmodernism were the critical reactions
to the old, established rhetoric's of recent human history, in its universality,
simplicity, and reductionism, and these 'posts' set out a flexible foundation for
the development of a 'posthuman culture' (Hassan, 1977), and arguably this
is continuing to take place.

Hassan might be credited by some as the first person to term 'posthumanism', but the past 50 years have seen many different versions of what
this concept might mean, exemplifying the challenges in trying to understand what 'human' is and what it might become. This can be seen in philosophical posthumanism and concepts that emerged from Haraway (Haraway,
1985), Hayles (1999), Gray with 'cyborg citizenship' (Gray, 2002), and works
around transhumanism by Bostrom (2002, 2003b), to more recent ideas from
Braidotti (2013) and Nayar (2014), all critiques of humanism, but in different ways. There are other ideas to contemplate too in these mind-blowing
debates about the 'human' and 'being' such as 'anti-humanism', but I take

some solace from Ferrando's (2012) 'statement' when summing up what 'posthumanism' can generally mean and how it connects to my reflections of being a critical community psychologist and thinking about marginalised people. For example, posthumanism challenges the anthropocentric humanism that dominates ideas, practices, and education in the West. Posthumanism therefore can also be about animals, artificial intelligence, and what might and does beyond our planet. This then suggests that posthumanism can be concerned with ecology and climate and not seeing the 'human' as top of a hierarchy above all things. These ideas resonate with me because they question not just what it means to be a 'human' or not, and what 'existence' means or not, but it opens up the possibilities of new ideas and perspectives in how we understand the most marginalised people and their contexts, not as a separate entity, but as something that is very much part of all of us in some way. It makes me think about the ideas that emerged relating to cyborgism (Haraway, 1985) and the transformation of biology developed around narratives of fear and uncertainty emerged, suggesting that despite the opportunities that are lauded about technological development, there are still insecurities about what living with machines or a cyborg might be like, if possible, without it threatening choices, personal autonomy, powers, and identities. This could be seen during the Covid-19 pandemic, where people were unsure about the use of digital technology and its use to communicate with people and to seek help and care for their medical conditions and for their mental health (see Anthony, 2021; Strudwick et al., 2021), but that is without ignoring the exacerbation of health and digital inequalities that others faced too who could not use, access or afford that technology to benefit (Davies et al., 2021).

Haraway's work on cyborgism, amongst other writers, however, was not so much concerned with the need to 'enhance' humanity, but instead picked at the traditional ideas of what it means to be human, which highlighted the social, cultural, historical, and political difficulties that this promotes. Haraway (1991) explored the fluid nature of the machine and its connection with living organisms, helping us to think about who we are now in times when our bodies can change through technological and digital interventions. Yes, it provides us with images of The Terminator from the film franchise (1984–2019) or Avatars or long dead singers appearing on stage as holograms, or even the singers of ABBA (famous pop band in the 1970s) appearing at concerts without being there, yet still very much alive. Yes, it invokes ideas of eternal life, strength, superhuman powers, and intelligence and magic and the power and control to change. But, beyond the transhumanist (or ultrahumanism, see Delio, 2012) and science fiction fantasies, there are clear realities that humans face. This is the important part of Haraway's ideas, and it is not so much whether we are robots or not, or whether we should expect Captain Kirk (from the film franchise Star Trek) to hover over earth in his spaceship, but that it inevitably rejects the humanist subject that we have known and has been established through Enlightenment ideals, hundreds of years ago. The cyborg, the terminator, the metaphor is really not about whether we will become a robot, instead it is the feminist underpinning to posthumanism that highlights the possibilities of what we can become. This rejects some of the offshoots of cyborgism and augmented humans such as perfectionism (body image and Instagram) and modifying one's body to create some form of 'perfectionism', a 'better' person, and for me, it has overtones of an 'ideal' human and 'normality', a self-actualisation that many can never live up to.

   This raises questions about equalities for marginalised people who cannot afford these modifications or are seen as the antithesis of reaching an 'ideal human' and may act as props for being something you *should not* be, underpinned by social, political, cultural, and historic influences. This is obvious in the lives of many excluded people, and this can be seen in the everyday nuances of communication, media, employment, and just going to the shops. Does the technology provide a life where what we do is more efficient and productive (in line with neoliberal values) and really enhance people's lives? Does it allow people to live longer, but longer in misery and continued marginalisation? It raises questions as to how we live, work, and how our futures might look, and indeed, may enhance class and racial divides rather than technology that can bring people together to move forward and enhance their lives. Overall, 'transhumanism' is an aspect of posthumanism (some may disagree) that looks to enhance the human through technology means such as nanotechnology and genetic engineering. If enhancement takes place and has arguably been taking place for decades, this could lead to a 'posthuman race' and may lead to curing diseases and turning humans as we think we know them into super beings, what Young (2006:15) calls 'overcoming human limitations through reason, science and technology'. Maybe this is just the next way for humans to evolve to sustain and live as long as possible over the longest possible time, putting 'nature' in transhuman hands (Young, 2006).

   Some of this came alive vividly with the onset of Covid-19 in 2020, where more use of Facebook, Twitter, MS Teams, and Zoom for people to communicate through laptops, mobile phones, and watches took place. Also, other technologies developed further such as lifestyle devices to monitor fitness. For example, 'smart pills' have been used to equip people with ingestible electronic sensors that track patients' compliance to medication (see Saher and Anjum, 2021). These technologies are digitalised approaches to control and care for people patients and other people, a form of disease management, through monitoring and surveillance. Even drones were used in places to disinfect places alongside robots who monitored aspects of social distancing as well as aiding some surgery and related procedures (see Kaiser et al., 2021). All this raises the same questions of the past on whether 'robots' are replacing 'humans' or are the humans controlling the robots and in effect robots are just a 'new' human or 'posthuman'. Maybe the use of drones and robots helped to ensure, to some extent, less human interaction to prevent the spread of disease and technological wearables like making use of Bluetooth and GPS technology, and helped to efficiently monitor some people's health, with a view to helping them, and added to a growing field of 'telemedicine'. Does this underpin the newer medical paradigm that is not just drug orientated and increasingly now reliant on technology and devices that can be controlled from afar? To some, this is a positive way forward for humans, has many people used technology through the Covid-19 pandemic to communicate with one another, to pass on information quickly, to help and support and provide some access to healthcare services such as counselling, but this did not happen for all. Not all people can afford technology and some marginalised groups are not allowed the use of technology such as prisoners and people incarcerated because of their mental health. For people who do have access to digital technology, some now speak of 'system overload' and that the continued use of technology has helped to cause mental health issues (Cheshmehzangi et al., 2022). Technology, for people who can use it, afford it, and trusts it, can be something great, for others, it is redundant because the humans who make it have made it to reach human ideals that only suit certain groupings of people. Did Covid-19 highlight that technology only works to an extent? Did it make us different 'humans' than what we had known? Technology that is meant to enhance our lives, in the same way that medical models are promoted as being lifesaving, appears to be just as reliable and unreliable for marginalised people.

The hard sciences and Cartesian dichotomies of the past (and very present too) could not have anticipated the acceleration of how technology has developed in the past 150 years, and in even more so in recent decades, from bulky machines to downloading massive amounts of information on an app. That would suggest in itself that how we live in our day-to-day life and how our communities' function have changed, whether we are 'cyborged' or not. Transhumanist thinking emerged as a way to think about how humans have evolved by means of science and technology (see Cordeiro, 2014). A classic example might be comparing ourselves to an advanced robot, like in the Terminator films, implying that we have made machines into human forms, with advanced intelligences and strengths, standard human vs. robotic human, artificial intelligence. This connects with the idea that the biological evolution of the human race will be taken over by advanced genetic and implantable technologies that artificially go beyond the 'natural', evolutionary process. Yet, when we experience a global catastrophe like Covid-19, where people at every level of society are involved, regardless of how rich or powerful one is, it highlights how useful technology can be and how alienating it can be too, raising questions about our identities as humans and how we fit in the world around us, and questions our obsession that technology always provides answers and happiness.

Established beings to becomers – Deleuze and Guattari

Traditional humanistic understandings of 'human' have been considered to be closed off and self-contained, with established binaries between genders, races, disabilities, sexualities, and other identities (see Carlson et al., 2021), a long distance from the ever-in-flux ambiguities, multiple identities, sub-jectivities that a posthuman perspective can bring, decentring people to a less privileged place above or under other people (see works by Massumi, 1992; Gibson, 2006). This links in with Deleuze and Guattari's (1987) idea of 'assemblages' that relates to how something (subject) is not static and posi-tioned, but something that is constantly changing and reinterpreting in a way that I have queeried my identities. This suggests that there is a constant shift between the connectivities between all things, not just between people, and it can be technologies, objects, emotions, and contexts too (see Liddiard et al., 2019). All things are therefore arguably dynamic, intersect, and reconfigure, which helps to understand a word I have already used several times in this book and that is 'becoming'.

The ontology of 'becoming' suggests that something is not just always in flux, but it has some direction and can lean away from being fixed, and through assemblages, the process of becoming may be and influenced by many factors from the biological to the political to the psychological (see Fox & Alldred, 2017; Gibson et al., 2021). 'Becoming' is therefore a form of progres-sion that is not linear, can break away or redirect itself and is ambiguous with a degree of knowing and being affirming, whilst resisting set boundaries. For example, Fritsch (2010) explored how for disabled people, they are constantly intertwined with multiple assemblages because of the use of guide dogs, wheelchairs, or hearing aids and point out that the concept of assemblage can move our thoughts about disabilities towards something that is relational that influences all beings and move away from the normative able-bodied per-spective that is forced upon by others. This relates to Deleuze and Guattari's idea of 'becoming' because the body, our minds, and our contexts are rela-tional and affected by many things, and this idea destabilises what is deter-mined by others to be fixed and 'being' as opposed to what we are forever 'becoming'. The idea of becoming then suggests that we are not stabilised identities that remain the same, but dynamic, powerful, and diverse, dismiss-ing the presumed medicalised idea that we are defined and remain defined by what we are told we are to be. And, whilst we pride ourselves on being our individual self's, in fact, we are multiple identities and multiple assemblages that have a shared and ever-changing identity with everything around us, that we affect and what affects us. Assemblages are not centralised, they can be linear, bent, fragmented, animate, or inanimate and intense, meaning that who we are is fluid and within many things at different times and places. This links in with a new materialistic position that sees living things as being in a world that is relational, plural, open, complex, uneven, and cuts across dualis-tic dichotomies and boundaries between different worlds (social, nature, cul-tural, biological). Arguably, this is in the context of a post-anthropocentric and posthumanist context because humans are no longer the central focus of social enquiry and new materialist ontology is not in line with universalism and moves towards diversity and multiplicity that goes beyond the estab-lished dichotomies (see Braidotti, 2022). For example, the 'body' is a political embodiment that goes beyond the biology and pathology of being under a microscope. In essence, humans are constructed and built upon exclusions through close assemblage with animals and technology and the body can be a symbol of oppression because of its appearance, function, and cultural position in our thinking and the world around us, ensuring that thinking about the 'human' as pathology and psychology at an individual level of analysis is too simplistic and not intersectional with how people and the world become.

The posthuman and critical posthumanities

The idea of 'becoming' resonates with me when thinking about my own identities that I explored earlier in the chapter. I do not feel that I have ever been one person, established by one identity, but whilst people are giving me different labels for different reasons to establish my 'being' and what I should 'be', they are inadvertently providing me with multiple assemblages. These assemblages are influenced by different forces and ideas, ensuring that I am a relational, complex, and diverse identity or identities, and questioning the established idea of what a 'human' is because the most marginalised groups in society must also feel the same in their day-to-day lives. Braidotti (2013) pointed out that the traditional distinction between what we understand to be 'human' and, the 'posthuman', explores how posthuman thinking displaces the traditional humanistic unity of the person/subject and this goes someway to make sense of flexible and multiple identities. Braidotti's perspective of posthumanism recognises humans in all their diversities; and the 'posthuman' aims to deconstruct the rigidity and permanency of the notion of what being 'human' means. The human therefore can no longer be defined as a binary with being non-human and maybe never was anyway. The ideas of posthumanism place humans among and not above other humans (Braidotti, 2013; Goodley, 2014), and this makes sense in the context that the ideas of a 'posthuman' are influenced not simply by critics of humanism, but through multiple disciplines and perspectives, which according to Ferrando (2014) helps to redefine the notion of the 'human' stemming from onto-epistemological, scientific, and biotechnological developments.

　Braidotti has played a part in the development of 'critical posthumanities', and this stems from the ideas already touched upon alongside other developing ideas about the human. 'Critical posthumanities' is the overarching and becoming set of ideas that are diverse and uneven that help to continue to dismantle and explore what we mean by the 'human' and can be considered as an approach that blurs over the ideas of 'posthumanism' and 'posthuman' by both considering science fiction and scientific fact too (Herbrechter, 2013, 2017). From Herbrechter's perspective, critical posthumanism concerns going back to contextualising the past views of the posthuman and the powerful desire to escape what we think we have always known to be 'human'. This is an ever-changing, relatively new paradigm of thinking that does not just continue to challenge what 'human' means but it also considers the ever-changing contexts that living things reside in that are influenced by global economic challenges, war, pandemics, and continued environmental problems that earth is facing, alongside the ever more powerful digitalisation of life and biomedia, and the continued blurring's of relationships between non-human and human life forms. In other words, the Anthropocene and biopolitics continue to be deconstructed and are becoming increasingly informed by strengthening processes in bioart, new media, and digital post/humanities (see Henriksen et al., 2021; Vint, 2022). This theoretical foundation analyses how people have shaped their lifestyles in line with digitalisation and virtual reality, alongside the conflicting traditions relating to the establishment of humanism, which can provide insights into what we might become or are becoming and how psychology can link with this and what it can become. With critical posthumanities, it means different outlooks and perspectives on what becoming means, and this book will blur itself across those ideas and how best it can be adapted to inform, interrogate, and reimagine a psychology that lives in the moment and going forward.

Nayar – Critical humanisms and posthuman visions

There has not been much directly written about psychology and its connections with posthumanist or posthuman thinking (but do see works by Brinkmann, 2017; Burman, 2018; Whitehead, 2018; Tironi et al., 2022); however, since being introduced to posthuman ideas, I cannot help but think about the possibilities it could bring for psychology from my positioning as a critical community psychologist. Discussing critical posthumanist thinking inevitably brings into conversations ideas about 'human', 'behaviour', and 'mind', exactly what most psychologists are concerned with in their research and practices. I then posit that the connection between them is worth considering and worth exploring to see if new ideas, visions, and perspectives can emerge that might make for a healthy contribution to debates, and within a critical posthumanities relational and fuzzy framework, I have found Nayar's (2014) analysis of the critical posthumanism helpful too.

Thinking about this, alongside Braidotti's work, I have found Nayar's use of critical posthumanism a useful way for psychologists of all kinds to think about the psychological aspects of advancements with technology. Also, Nayar posited that the changing ideological positions and diversities of human might help to reconsider traditional humanistic ideals and the politics that sets out humans from other forms of life as exclusionary, something that should concern all kinds of psychologists. Nayar (2014:8) points out that 'critical posthumanism' concerns that:

1   The human is co-evolving and shares everything from ecosystems to life processes with all life forms including animals.
2   Technology is an integral part to human identity.

Nayar suggested that critical posthumanism makes the connection between humanism's (traditional) exclusionary practices and claims that the exclusion- ary nature of being a 'human' is where we can find the origins of oppressive practices that exclude people (also see Richards, 2015b). This helped me to reflect back on my time working in the community with marginalised peo- ple and critically examine the central concept and approach that seemed to unite all professionals, that being 'person-centred' or 'person-centred care', which invokes ideas of inclusion, empowerment, and participation at equal levels with marginalised people, but it was never clear-cut that this was actu- ally happening. It also reminded me of my first introduction to Marx and the idea of the 'opium of the people' in relation to religion, and I felt this was the same for how professionals, experts, and the structures they work in are completely convinced that 'person-centredness' is for the good of every- one, particularly in social care and who are excluded by society. There was never a sense of co-evolving, but more ameliorative and tokenistic attempts to 'person-centred care' that ensured voices were minimal or non-existent. It was always 'Other', and 'Other' was enshrined within complex power tussles between people who needed care, and ambitious professionals and leaders who could be domineering and egotistical, underpinned by funder and fund- ing expectations that needed outcomes that were usually numerical. I will discuss some of these issues as I develop the narrative in the book, but Nayar and Braidotti's ideas around critical posthumanities helped me to think crit- ically about this presumed framework of 'person-centredness', which seemed at odds with how people were developing and becoming. There is a lack of critical analysis of 'person-centredness' and it seems to me that it continues to be a guise for the real flaws that ensured exclusionary practices that top-down person-centredness can bring. A critical posthumanities outlook for me was useful because it was concerned with not just being a binary between human- ism and anti-humanism or person-centred vs. not person-centred that encap- sulates the ideologies around social care in the UK, but instead it felt like a 'discourse of life', which connected the complications, impurities, mutuality, and multiple distinctiveness's of life, a life that is about 'becoming' through new connections between all life forms and technologies (see Nayar, 2014).

With critical posthumanism concerning 'co-evolvement', which is symbiotic and becoming with all other species, it is then concerned with the intercon- nections and mergers with other genes and life forms that ensure human existence, meaning we all count at lots of fuzzy levels of power and intercon- nection. Nayar (2014) calls this posthuman thinking a 'companion species' in which we form a multispecies citizenship, a 'species cosmopolitan' and this is connected to a 'posthuman biology' and 'symbiogenesis' (a sense of becoming by living together). This helps to consider life in different ways because technological changes have ensured that life is different, and this could be a useful way to think about 'person-centredness' in health and social care or psychology's poor record, for example, in promoting the importance of climate change because it affects all living things, and our behaviours are strongly related to how this emerges (see Trott et al., 2022). Nayar makes the point that we live in a 'biological state' which excludes the personal, the cultural, the historical, our affiliations, and our identities, but also explained that 'pedagogy' relating to the fact that the species cosmopolitan needs to 'learn' and that pedagogy is central to survival, and to evolution in a species cosmopolitan.

The merger of genes and learning is what can keep the species cosmopolitan going and through this a 'posthuman citizenship', which incorporates the mathematised, biologically producing body with the co-evolvement with other life forms and technology would be beneficial for all, all of which is connected to the political, cultural, spiritual, and social influences of our becoming. For example, biometrics and the body are an example of how the body has changed, meaning that the body and 'human' must be considered as different than what has gone before (traditional humanism). The human is a 'node' that is reliant on other forms of life, genetics, information for its continued evolution, but that it is also about considering citizenship as embodied that interconnects with the environment (Nayar, 2014). The implications for psychology could be that the 'body' is not an objective organism that can be reduced to bit parts, like trying to understand a car stripped down and needing to put it together again when you are not a mechanic. Understanding human behaviour must be understood in the context of the human interaction with all life forms, technology, and biology. Maybe if the multiple strands of psychology worked more collectively rather than as separated psychologies, and psychologies that are sold as different psychologies, a new identity in psychology could develop that embraces both the individual and individual in rhizomatic contexts.

Whilst a cynic would suggest that the idea of a species cosmopolitan seems like we would be living on a planet where it is like 'the Planet of the Apes' (1968/2011) or 'Waterworld' (1995) (futuristic Hollywood films) or another Marvel film, where we are just fighting for survival or having dinner at a restaurant with a colony of ants or a real life 'Tiger Who Came to Tea' (Kerr, 1968), a 'companion species' would mean an appreciation of not just biology and technology but of the cultural, political, social, historical and multiple identities that make us who we are, something that is lacking in psychology. When thinking about the 'brain' or human behaviour, we must always be thinking, what encompasses these things together, rather than seeing separate parts. Humans, and our relations with other humans and living organisms, must be beneficially mutual and not exclusionary, and climate change is a good example of the significance of this idea. Posthumanism mostly rejects the established binaries and autonomous subjectivity, which we are inclined to apply to our understanding of human behaviour, and is more orientated towards a developing cosmopolitan of species that is intersectional and becoming. This idea calls for us to respect the multiple and diverse nature and nurture of what it means to be human and all things, which is the crux of a critical posthumanities outlook for me.

Summary

The chapter began with a frank opening of some of the discrimination my dad, family, and I have faced over the decades. This was not to try to portray myself as a victim or to find empathy, but it was a reflection that highlighted my own challenges of working out who I am or who we are in ever-changing contexts alongside ever-changing 'humans', which raises questions about my/our identities and relationships with people. I provided a relatively brief overview of the development of 'posthumanism' and the 'posthuman'. Brief, because there are so many nuances, theories, perspectives, frustrations, and uneven territories that could not be covered all in one go, all in one small book, and the broad-brush strokes of examples and ideas are just providing some initial thoughts for the rest of the book, rather than regurgitating the whole literature on posthumanism. This chapter aimed to tease out some views and ideas that have emerged that are not often directly talked about in the context of psychology, and so my limited and narrow focus on a couple of perspectives and ideas is just one way to raise questions and reflections to start that conversation, in line with the queerying nature of the narrative.

The chapter sets the scene from some angles of posthumanism in terms of understanding the 'human' (if it exists), and whether we have maybe always been posthuman, if we are always in flux, in all its complexities and starts to lay down the roots that start to consider psychology's place within those debates. For the rest of this book, the narrative will connect with posthuman and critical posthuman perspectives to guide an analysis that reflects on psychology's place and identities. There will be a dipping in and out of the ideas that have emerged from Braidotti and Nayar's works, but other aspects of posthumanism will be connected too, acknowledging the ambiguous and changing nature of humans and theories and ideas relating to the human. This might provide a more open-minded reflection on what 'psychology' means in the 21st century, and what it might become.

2 Psychology – Stuck in the past or a becoming psychology?

I noted in Chapter 1 that the history of posthumanism and the developing field of critical posthumanities is made up of many different views and disagreements about what it means to be human. This is mainly because humans have changed and have kept changing, ensuring that we are complicated and diverse human beings that are forever in flux and open to many interpretations, and within and around us, the world changes too, at cosmos, political, historical, social, cultural, and discursive levels. But what about psychology's place in all this? As a chartered psychologist and critical community psychologist, it is no surprise that when thinking about what it means to be a human and how we might understand that in the context of disabled people and other marginalised groups, that you wonder about psychology's place within those ontologies. After all, a general and common definition of psychology states that psychology is the scientific study of the human mind and behaviour, and the study of psychology has become increasingly powerful and popular in recent decades, in its many forms and perspectives. In this respect, the very study of psychology is all about the 'human' for what we think it is or not and therefore, an interrogation is needed of this discipline to consider where our understandings of humans are and where it could go.

To begin to think about psychology's place within conversations about what it means to be human, the chapter will briefly review the development of modern psychology over the past 150 years to provide an overview of the structural make-up of mainstream psychology and what it has become or not in the present day. This means picking and choosing bits of history to help inform the central narrative rather than trying to cover the whole history of psychology. In Chapter 1, I briefly examined that the concept of 'human' cannot remain static and that our identities are ambiguous, subjective, and a series of assemblages that are constantly changing, reinterpreting, and intersecting with many things. If this is the case, then a discipline like psychology or 'mainstream psychology', you would expect to also be constantly in flux, ambiguous, and diverse. Additionally, I considered the ontological viewpoint of 'becoming' a progressive and non-linear way of breaking away from static and fixed positions to something that is affirming and boundary resistant (Deleuze & Guattari, 1987). This fits in with a new materialist

DOI: 10.4324/9781003057673-2

and vitalist position that sees living things as plural and relational that is not just 'human' focused based on old humanistic tiered values, but one that is multiple, diverse, and beyond set binaries (Braidotti, 2013). The chapter will then think about some of these key points from critical posthumanities and consider how relevant this could be for psychology and whether it might help us to consider mainstream psychology, as a psychology that can emerge and develop into a continuous and 'becoming' psychology that can decentre itself to something marginalised people can connect with.

Psychology lecture with a difference

I was once asked to deliver a lecture to a group of about 100 psychology undergraduates in a large lecture theatre. The topic of the lecture was around 'intelligence', a classic and traditional theme in the teaching of undergraduate psychology in the UK. My work at the time outside of the university involved working with a group of adults with intellectual disabilities, and we had spent lots of time talking about what 'intelligence' meant to them and we questioned the meaning of this word and how it is interpreted in scientific terms.

I invited the group of men and women to the lecture that I was due to deliver to the psychology students. The plan was to not just introduce the concept of 'intelligence' to the students but to get them to think about this in a critical way. I asked the students and the group of people I invited to complete an IQ test. This was a surprise to everyone, especially for the group of people invited because some were not able to read or write and all of them had not studied beyond college courses in the local area. However, what was important was not completing the test and seeing how well they might have done, but more about how they felt about doing this and whether it was a good way to help understand their intelligence and the intelligence of others. The students and group of adults were eager to engage and test themselves.

The feeling in the lecture theatre once the test was done was what you would expect in any examination room once an exam is complete, and that is complete relief. Despite the relative informality of it all, the mindset for the students was that this was an exam, and 'I must do well in it', whereas the group of people invited, felt lost and uncomfortable with the whole process, but persevered knowing what the plan was to be for the rest of the lecture.

Are IQ tests the best way to determine whether someone is of high 'intelligence'?

After a break, I asked the students to listen to two performances that were to be delivered by the group invited. The first performance was a short play, created and performed by the group, about their experiences of being labelled with intellectual disabilities, and the second performance was by one man who wanted to share his poetry about love, life, and sexuality (see Richards, 2017). The group had previously done similar work for an advocacy project, and they were prepared and had practised to deliver their work to the students.

The performances that were presented proved to be a powerful way to critically examine the meaning of intelligence and what life was like for disabled people. The reaction of the students in the audience was emotional that led to some crying, some were happy, some were sad, and for others, it left questions about what intelligence means in the context of how we understand disabilities.

The performances were followed up with a group discussion about intelligence in the context of reason, logic, and mathematics that underpins an IQ test and the creative performances in the context of the power of the arts and voice to share expertise and experiences. The debates were energised and thought-provoking. It was a revelation to the students that intelligence was more than just an examination to test how much you know, but intelligence can be anything.

The makings of the 'human mind' – God and soul

The vignette suggests that we should consider 'intelligence' as something that is relational, emotional, varied, and vivid alongside something that might be scientific, mathematical, and logical. The students were studying for a British Psychological Society accredited degree in the UK, where the 'cornerstones' of psychology are centralised as the most important, such as clinical, counselling, forensic, and neuropsychology over lesser taught psychologies such as critical, political, and cultural psychologies, limiting the teaching of psychology to something simple, specific, and definitive (see British Psychological Society, 2022). However, when the students opened up to a provocative discussion about what intelligence means from the perspective of a marginalised group, a group who delivered a creative take on intelligence, the students were challenged, and their minds were opened to a psychology of difference beyond the simplification of people they were more familiar with in an experiment that might assess intelligence and behaviour.

The reality is that when you explore the concept of 'intelligence' within the study of psychology, you are presented with a reductionist and linear epistemology of what 'intelligence' is and should be, that some might describe as 'psychobabble' because a post-truth psychology presents itself as something that can be relied upon, even when one psychologist says one thing, and another psychologist can say something completely different (Palmer, 2016; Hughes, 2018). But this is not a surprise because much of the psychology that we know today primarily concerns that psychology is a 'scientific' discipline and that human behaviour can only be understood properly through systematic processes and experimental measures to understand the way the 'human' thinks and behaves. Therefore, it 'must' be reliable and correct, and this is remarkable considering how new psychology is in the context of time. Through most of history, Western and Eastern ideas and philosophies were primarily enshrined in how divine forces make us how we are, not science and experimentation that makes up much of the identity of psychology today. Most of these divine ideas suggested that we have a 'soul' that was created by God, giving our bodies and lives a sense of purpose, with our bodies interconnected with our souls and minds (Brett, 1921/2013). To some degree, the 'human soul' was not just connected to our bodies but it was also in some way programmed and controlled, and our thoughts were known by God, which results in how we behave and interact with the world around us. Indeed, for many people, this belief is still important and a part of their lives that should be respected, and this is an important part of their identities in the present, but science was to gradually squeeze these ideas out of the thinking systems about what makes or made us human.

As philosophies, sciences, and ideas developed over the centuries, different explanations for 'human' and 'human behaviour' emerged. For so long, to understand the 'human' and 'human behaviour', a primary aim of understanding behaviour was that God was seen as the 'governor' of all things. That has included ideas and eternal truths that 'he' alone knows and without God, we would not have them, and this connects to Berkeley's 'idealism', that can be interpreted as whatever we think and do, it is caused by God (see King et al., 2013). To know God then was to know 'eternal truths', including what is bad or good, right, or wrong or what is beautiful or not, and this could not be changed because this was absolute. This is problematic because we all have fantasies, bad thoughts alongside the good thoughts, whatever good or bad is anyway, so to say this reflects the thoughts of God seems unusual, and that idealism was powerful, and in many respects, the established and dominant religions of our world still maintain aspects of that idealism, and for some, defines who they are, or what they will become and hope to become. But this links in with the ideas of Augustine and Aquinas (see Schumacher, 2011) later and they were of the view that divine intervention helps us to see intellectually what truth is and through this process, people will be happier and live a good life. This kind of philosophical position also implied that reason and our connection to God is the way to find truth and therefore answers questions about who we are, linking cognitive functioning with faith and God.

Whilst these ideas that will be familiar to many and will seem logical to some, it would also suggest that this makes for a complex relationship between being rational, reasoned, and at the same time connected with God, even more so if you have different religious and spiritual beliefs. This makes me think that whereas much is currently being written about what it means to be human, across many disciplines, it is a process that has continuously taken place through history. Humans are always asking the questions 'who am I?' and 'What is my place in the world or universe'? For some, and for a large part of history, the answer to this was God or Gods, and for many, that is still the case in their belief systems today. However, the divine stranglehold on humanity in some form or another was challenged, and the rationalism that came with the links with God and understanding eternal truths have been turned into science. A rationalism that cuts out a God, with God being taken over by science, or at least both started to compete with one another for truth and control of what being a human means, and this is still apparent in much of Western society today and beyond.

Modern psychology – From God to the lab

With the emergence of modern science, scientific psychology, and therefore the beginnings of the contemporary psychology, many have come to know when they first start to learn about psychology today, psychology started to become established in the 19th century. Many who have undertaken a psychology degree in the UK/the West will know that when they first start studying this discipline they are taught that psychology began in 1879 at the University of Leipzig, directed by Wilhelm Wundt. From this point (if that is your starting point for psychology), other departments and laboratories started to open in the Western world with a view to analyse human behaviour, from a scientific perspective. However, it is worth noting that there were a number of precursors that led up to Wundt's psychology laboratory that arguably informs the underpinning principles of modern psychology and aspects of contemporary/mainstream psychology today. For example, the British Associationalists, and Hartley who is often considered a founder to this group of people, related the brain and nerves to particles that vibrated and that this connects to thought (see Craig, 2020). Alongside this and his fellow Associationalists was the idea that similarity led to association, a forerunner to the ideas that would later emerge in learning theories and behaviourism. Around the same time, James and John Mills emerged with their ideas of human behaviour. Mills senior, an advocate for the 'brick-wall hypothesis', suggested that the mind should be considered a machine, like Locke's *table rasa*, meaning that our experiences are linked to ideas that form. Mills junior, on the other hand, felt that human nature was governed by forces yet to be found and understood (see Hyland, 2020). Either way, these conversations have a feel of a 'nature vs. nurture' debate that you have with students or colleagues at work in the present, and these thoughts were also debated years ago seemingly questioning the human and human behaviour, always directly or indirectly asking 'what is human' and what we become and what we mean in the context of life and Earth.

The other precursors that emerged before Wundt that have a connection to the history of psychology, included the development of 'psychophysics', that considered the relationship between the physical and psychological, and other developments such as physiognomy that linked personality with how your face looks (if you look nice, you must be nice) and phrenology (Gall 1758–1828) where it was hypothesised that the brain was responsible for mental faculties, and some parts of the brain were bigger than others, so associated to bumps on the skull. Essentially, if you read the lumps, you read the mind. Compared to today's analysis of personalities, faces and shapes of skulls, this seems absurd, but is it so far-fetched to say that people do not judge faces with expected personalities today? We only need to look at the Big Brother type reality television programmes that are broadcast constantly to see that this is what people do, even with no reasoned or objective scientific evidence to back this up, if indeed that is needed to judge someone anyway. Furthermore, it was not just the face that was being aligned with personality and behaviour, body shapes were also linked to personality. Galton and Binet (see Collins, 1999), for example, connected physical appearance with mental deficiencies, and this physiognomist perspective was taken further with Sheldon's take on humans having three body shapes and each shape is connected to a specific temperament (see Pailhez & Bulbena, 2010). Whilst many of these ideas are now laughed at and are discredited, we still hear people talk about personality in relation to bodily appearance, and we still make behavioural associations about the height and weight of people and how they might behave and respond to the world around them (see the Body Image Movement, 2012, a movement that inspires people to embrace their bodies).

Other forerunners to modern psychology started to emerge as well including, Helmholtz and sensory psychophysiology, where links were made with nerve impulses/sensory nerves in humans and used touch as a stimulus to understand decision making and movement. In the later Victorian period, EEG and fMRI emerged with the use of electric currents running through the brain and detected through electrodes through the scalp (see Chung & Hyland, 2012), and this will be familiar to many readers because they have experienced this themselves in some way or will know somebody who has experienced these processes. So, much of the forerunning ideas before Wundt's laboratory emerged were very much based on the assumption that there is a physiological basis for the minds that we have and develop and this could be understood only through scientific and experimental methods, through a process of observation and linear judgement. Therefore, it is no surprise that Wundt and the people who developed other psychology laboratories after him and beyond have to some degree followed a similar pattern in that they link the physiology of our bodies, especially the brain, with behaviour, dismissing the influences of the body and mind that are amalgamated in political, social, cultural, and economic influences.

Wundt and beyond

With Wundt often referred to as the 'father of experimental psychology' or the 'first psychologist', it ensures that the modern psychology that started then would have a foundation that was going to be scientific, reductionist, and pathological in nature when understanding the human and human behaviour, sharp contrasts to the critical posthumanity ideas that have been discussed in Chapter 1 and how psychology was to develop and become diverse in the later 20th century. The structuralist approach Wundt took to understanding thought and its subsequent behaviour was introspective in that it focused on the sensory processes or low-level perceptual process that influenced behaviour. Chung and Hyland (2012) however, do point out that he was also interested in 'volkerpsychologie', a 'folk psychology' where Wundt wrote about, for instance, that to understand ethics then, customs and beliefs need to be studied, which as an ethnographic feel to it, a far cry from the experimental psychology that most will be familiar with. Nevertheless, the reductionist approach to understanding humans was only to strengthen and be at the core of mainstream psychology over the next 100 years in ways that resonate with Hobbes materialist approach (see Springborg, 2016) that humans are like engines, so human behaviour can be explained by the individual body and the causes operating it. Meaning that souls do not exist, and we are governed by biological forces, and this idea influenced work around human perception, attention and concentrating, human thoughts, dreams and imagination, that were to become central and core themes that are still at the heart of 21st century psychology across associations, practices, and psychology departments in universities and beyond.

Around the same time that modern psychology was establishing itself in the West, Darwin's theory of evolution was emerging and becoming a dominant, scientific paradigm that remains today in the 21st century. In his book 'The Origin of Species', Darwin refers to the evolution of the mind and he felt the mind emerged like all other characteristics through natural evolution, with humans having an advantage over an animal promoting the Anthropocene. William James's ideas about psychology became established in his 'Principles of Psychology' (1890), with his views based on observation rather than experimentation. A key tenet of his views was that the mind evolved because it has a function to do, and therefore as humans evolved, the mind became more important. The physiological basis of human behaviour continued through the James-Lange theory of emotion (see Wassmann, 2010), suggesting that human experience of emotion comes from a physiological change that responds to external events and influences, a functionalist perspective that seeks to find causal relationships between internal thoughts and external behaviours. Whilst this seems encouraging that external influences are explored, it was still done in way that leaves out so much about who a person is and why they behave the way they do when interacting with the world around them, a far cry from the relationality of different critical posthumanity perspectives.

It seems that in those early days of modern psychology, psychology/psychologists were trying to work out what psychology was, and this seems to be the case in many respects now. Is psychology a science? Can psychology only be understood in scientific and reductionist terms? With so many psychologies within psychology today, the biological through to the political, is psychology too complex to be called 'psychology'? Does this indicate that psychology is a new materialist phenomenon that it will not admit too because if there are many psychologies, has it already become relational, plural, open and demonstrates its unevenness and many grey areas, maybe it was inevitable that with such a rigid and linear science based history that it would have to become something that is more relational and diverse. Yet, the universalist and centring nature of psychology, obsessed with binaries, remains dominant in psychology as ever before and this can be seen in powerful psychologies like clinical and forensic psychology.

For instance, we might think of Galton and Binet as historical figures in psychology who developed intelligence testing and IQ tests, but in essence, they are still applied in the same way well into the 21st century. These psychologists with others were very much followers of Social Darwinism (Albee, 1996), taking concepts like natural selection and survival of the fittest and applied this to humans and their intelligence. This ensured that intelligence/ IQ was viewed as an innate quality, with people with low IQ's considered weaker, which is a weak assumption in the context of the vignette earlier in the chapter, and yet powerful enough to ensure that, for example, disabled people will be excluded from schools, workplaces, and positions of power in government to this very day. The eugenics movement of the 1920s used Social Darwinism to advocate the separation of the weak minded from the strong minded, ensuring that already marginalised groups were further marginalised (see Winfield, 2012). Are we still seeing this today in how and who is treated within the mental health systems? Is it exclusively only marginalised groups who tend to fall into psychologised categories of 'deviant', 'less intelligent', and 'weak'? It seems that the spine of today's mainstream psychology is underpinned by values that would be familiar to psychologists from a hundred years ago, ensuring that psychology has somehow remained the same even that it many ways we understand it to be different today because of the advancements of technology, ideas, and attitudes. Yet, the development of mainstream psychology and other psychologies could also mean that psychology is already an example of a posthuman psychology, but underpinned by traditional medical models of control, defining, being powerful and controlling, suggesting that psychology is an identity crisis.

Further into the 20th century, most psychologists would have described themselves as behaviourists. The image that might spring to mind is rats in laboratories, after all, the roots of behaviourism are in animal research because the assumption is that animals are easier to study than humans and that comparisons can be made (see Logue, 1985). For example, Pavlov in Russia examined animals and tested behaviour using dogs, leading to the well-known ideas relating to unconditioned stimulus and conditioned responses, resulting in a form of conditioning. Similar, Watson in the USA was developing work around similar ideas and he posited that all behaviour is learned from the environment, but that psychology should be seen as a science that reports in a way that is empirical and controlled, and that there is not much difference between the learning of humans and in animals. Whilst behaviourist psychology is no longer the dominant paradigm within psychology, it still plays a part in the underpinning ideas that are connected to association learning that still influence clinical and educational practice, still leaving today's psychology with a clear link to a scientific and experimental past that you now see in different forms in neuropsychology and cyberpsychology. The simplicity of experiments and statistics, a reduction of who someone might be, rejects the possibilities of diversity and complex identities that a critical posthumanities perspective would promote.

It is prudent to note that even before the behaviourists laid their roots in the developing modern psychology, that Freud, Jung, and others were also developing their theories, and like some behaviourist thinking, still plays a major part in contemporary psychology and beyond today, and dominates many parts of modern Western thinking (see Parker, 2022). Ironically, Freud was not a psychologist, but more a therapist, and yet, his connection with psychology is profound and complicated. Psychology was not particularly concerned with mental illness, for example, and neither was it focused on therapy, but whatever way you look at it, Freud's ideas aimed to explore and change behaviour, and this is important because those ideas relate to power, difference, decision making, choice, and inclusion and cannot be ignored. There is not a semester that goes by in class with my students where I have to explain that 'psychoanalysing' is not about profiling a criminal, and instead it goes much deeper in someways and simplistic in other ways, and how we understand the 'structure of the mind' cannot be determined with simplistic experiments in a laboratory (depending on what you believe). Freud's ideas of the psychosexual stages of development or dream analysis or defence mechanisms, however, have raised questions about humans and their behaviour, maybe in a way that had never been done, and plenty of psychodynamic theorists were to follow ranging from Jung, Erikson, Horney, Klein, and his own daughter Anna Freud, who would challenge his views and take those ideas to other places in exploring 'humankind'.

The book is not here to cover the whole history of Freud, or psychology, alongside all the other protagonists in modern psychology's history, and the wider and deeper historical roots of psychoanalysis, but Freud's philosophies did help to develop psychology further and go beyond, to some extent, the laboratories filled with rats. Freud was searching for answers to what made up a human, albeit primarily at an individualised level. His work remains controversial and challenging, and the emergence of logical positivists and Popper's (2002) falsification principles undermined some of Freud's ideas because they were unfalsifiable, and indeed, Wittgenstein (see Harcourt, 2016) proposed that psychoanalysis is not a science and Grünbaum (1986) said that psychoanalytical theories of any kind are difficult to test empirically. The analysis here could go further about what positives, negatives, and opportunities there are for Freud's theories and the theories that have developed from him since, but whatever way you view it, he questioned what humans were about and asked questions about what makes us who we are, albeit from a reductionist perspective, but in a way like never before, and that is something that has to keep happening because of the ambiguous and becoming ways of human-hood and all things.

Humanism, existentialism, and phenomenology

Am I human?

Odd, strange, genius, inspiring, awkward, difficult, quiet, annoying, loud, stubborn, evil, lovely, complex, simple, terrible, nice.

Whether it be my family, schoolteachers, workplaces from managers or colleagues, relationships or lovers or my general social life, all the words above have been used to describe me, in all sorts of intersubjective contexts and situations, direct or indirectly, on paper or on screen or face-to-face. This would suggest that I must be the most complex human being that has ever existed, indeed, maybe I am not human, or human as we think we know it.

My reflections on the adjectives above are if that is how people in different times and different places have viewed me then I must have experienced multiple assemblages, I must be relational, dynamic, and non-binary.

Somehow, despite the multifaceted 'being' that has been established about me by different people in their different contexts, I have managed to be successful, build a career, own a house, drive a car, be a parent, a traveller, a writer, and be privileged albeit that has come through lots of hard work and luck.

Now, think about these words again.

Odd, strange, genius, inspiring, awkward, difficult, quiet, annoying, loud, stubborn, evil, lovely, complex, simple, terrible, nice.

In the same contexts, in day-to-day life and within established societal institutions, I have heard similar words being used to describe disabled people alongside their other marginalised identities such as being different ethnicities, genders, classes, and sexualities.

With those adjectives and labels, alongside the label of 'disabled', disabled people do not find themselves in a privileged position that I have found myself in. They are less likely to build a career, own a house, drive a car, be a parent, a traveller, and a writer.

Why is it different for me without an established label of disability compared to disabled people? We are all human, but we are not the same?

Whilst Freud problematised issues that people face mostly in relation to their childhoods or something that relates to a 'conscious', at the turn of the 20th century, other ideas started to emerge through postmodernism and poststructuralism, and the developments of humanistic philosophies of existentialism and phenomenology, meant that our analysis of 'human' was increasingly becoming complex when analysing this issue. My reflections above consider myself as someone who is perceived to be different and multi-faceted, but somehow, I have bypassed the issues that disabled people face to a neoliberal position of money, education, and status, and yet I am no different in terms of identities and all the ambiguities that come with being human. It raises questions of existence, experience, and how societies are structured and emerge around people. These kinds of ideas emerged from existentialists, phenomenologists, and humanists and all have in some form, or another have a concern with improving wellbeing of people, and these ideas of existentialism and phenomenology are broadly connected to the 'humanistic psychology' that started to be formed earlier in the 20th century, and we can see these kinds of reflective processes at the very heart of psychologies such as counselling psychology today.

The dominant names and many of their ideas from the emergence of humanistic psychology of the 1950s is still powerful today. At the heart of humanistic person-centredness and psychologies that connect themselves to a 'humanistic psychology', are the ideals of Maslow's 'hierarchy of needs' and Rogers for his ideas around self-worth and conditional and unconditional positive regard (see Arnold & Foncubierta, 2021). Both, in contrast, to the key ideas of the other paradigms dominating psychology in the late 19th and early 20th centuries, believed that people should strive for a self-actualisation to strive for the person we really are, and that a free, subjective, and unique self can develop towards a genuine and authentic self, instead of becoming what we told we should become. These ideas alongside other humanistic thinkers of those times are very much influenced by the traditions of existential and phenomenological traditions of the time and past 150 years and much earlier in some cases. For example, Kierkegaard, a founder of existentialism, suggested that one should view the construction of systems by expressing one's own existence within that individual, so for that person to decide their own existence and to examine it rather than someone else doing it for you from an objective stance (see Mehl, 2010), ideas that resonate with today's humanistic psychology and person-centred approaches.

In the context of humanistic psychology, it grew out of the rejection of behaviourism and psychoanalysis and became known as the 'third force'. The aim was that people should be able to find meaning in their own lives, which meant talking about their lives and their identities rather than this being judged in an objective way that led to personal growth (like Rogers Ideas), different from being in a therapy that focuses on mental illness, meaning that humanistic psychology was for all, not just people who had mental health issues (Hoffman et al., 2020). However, at the same time, drug therapy started to emerge, and the onset of the development of anti-psychotic and anti-depressant medication was revolutionary and ensured that the medical model of mental health and how behaviour was understood enhanced its power. The quick fixes and feelings of being 'cured' in effect challenged the approach of personal growth and reaching self-actualisation because for some, without drug interventions, they would not feel that they could reach their potential, even that drug therapy had its drawbacks with side effects and dependency. Drug therapy might have helped some with some symptoms, but it was not a cure and was more likely to control behaviour in a way that was inappropriate or changed their identities (see Richert, 2019).

The cultural revolution of the 1960s was in part to influence the development of the anti-psychiatry movement and rejection of the medical authority to control and dictate how someone was diagnosed and treated, whilst other civil rights movements were also emerging fighting for rights for black people, gay people, and other marginalised groups in society (see Murray, 2014). 'Voice' was as important as ever in promoting identities and people who wanted to look beyond the narrowed vision of psychologised and medicalised models of mental health and human behaviour in general. Some of the protests, ideas, and provocations of this time heavily influenced other branches of psychology that started to emerge as a counterattack to the established order within psychology that was inherently scientific and medical in nature and how it viewed people such as community psychology. Yet, the individualistic nature of humanistic psychology was still an issue because people were being decontexualised and in doing so were being depoliticising, so further ideas emerged that brought these issues to wider attention.

Qualitative, social constructionism, and critical psychology

With decontexualising and depoliticising being an issue, the ideas of 'social constructionism' started to establish in the 1960s (Berger & Luckmann, 1966), which suggests that our realities are socially constructed rather than constructed by individuals alone, meaning that our realities come from social interaction, not in isolation. This means that our social realities can be considered through discourses of conversations between people, and from a methodological point of view, qualitative analysis then allows an analysis of language that provides a deeper meaning of a reality that is not so easy using quantitative methods (see Burr, 2015). Some of the ideas that emerged from this can also be seen in the 'crisis in social psychology' that emerged in the 1970s. Gergen (1973) for instance challenged the experimental approaches of social psychologists that ignored cultural and historical factors that shape behaviour, with social actions not being static that can be simply observed because they are fluid and ever-changing. Similarly, Israel and Tajfel (1972) called for psychologists to look beyond experimentation as a way to understand people and to open up a dialogue with other disciplines and other countries beyond the domination of North American psychology. In other words, these authors, amongst others, wanted change on how social psychology was formed and what methods were used. Indeed, from here, more qualitative methods started to be employed in psychology, but the teaching, research and practice of psychology was and still remains dominated by quantitative methods and analyses. This is because for psychologists to measure, observe, and provide logical conclusions to their work, quantitative methods align with that very well, whereas qualitative methods that might incorporate diaries, conversations, arts such as drama and poetry, cause disruption in a way that challenges the powerful status quo. This radical disruption could also be seen in discourse analysis and interpretative phenomenological analysis, which emerged as ways to understand the language and experiences of others, helping to think about people in context (see Willig, 2015). In effect by doing so, it was questioning and re-understanding what it means to be human; however, this has not had the radical effect on psychology that these analyses had hoped for and have only had a partial impact in the broader dimensions of mainstream psychology.

But that did not stop and prevent other 'new' psychologies such as 'critical psychology' from emerging. It goes without saying that 'critical' psychology is a psychology that is not happy with what psychology was, is, and what it became and still is today. Critical psychologists in general emerged because like some social constructionists, they wanted to see a psychology that felt more humane and had deeper meaning, completely the opposite to the positivist and quantitative ways of psychology (see Gough et al., 2013; Burr, 2015). And, maybe more importantly, and what sets it out to be different from other forms of psychology, is that it is concerned with power and the political, and that this is central to psychology, but mainstream psychology as a discipline essentially ignores the powerful and political manifestations that encompass psychology. This then ensures that there are unfair and unequal relationships, which resonates with Marxist perspectives around capitalism and neoliberalism. This can also be seen in critical psychology's rejection of the rise of conservatism and republicanism that dominated the 1980s, driven by Reganism and Thatcherism in the USA and UK. Sadly, critical psychology is not something that is a core part of many psychology curriculums in universities, maybe in the same way that you do not see sociology much in schools because both disciplines seek to challenge the status quo and challenge systems of power that infiltrate not just psychology, but all that psychology influences.

Contemporary psychology – UK and beyond

The emergence of psychologies that were critical or community orientated in nature, with strong qualitative and creative backdrops, and their influences on university programmes and research, however, has not been transformative in my view. The contemporary psychology we know that has developed over the past 150 years is underpinned by post-positivism, logical empiricism, and falsification, ensuring that the lens of mainstream psychology is mostly focused on reality being observed, tested, and established through scientific methods (Leahey, 1992; Botha, 2021). This means that mainstream psychology represents something that is mostly value-free and separated from cultural, political, social, and economic influences and any notion that it could engage with a critical posthumanities way of thinking that views people as assemblages or a cosmopolitan that is connected with all things, is not likely to be greeted with any favour, unless in-roads are made across psychology and other disciplines.

The positivist outlook of mainstream psychology is linked with essentialist and medical models that promote normalisation and distinctions between diversity and difference often with the latter presented in negative ways. This is disappointing because it feels like for all the progressive influences over the past 50 years, psychology is arguably the same as it ever was. For instance, The British Psychological Society in the UK (2022) posits that it aims to 'embrace equality, equity, diversity and inclusion' alongside being the 'authoritative and public voice of psychology', which seem contradictory, but then on another page the organisation defines 'psychology' as this:

> As a science psychology functions as both a thriving academic discipline and a vital professional practice, one dedicated to the study of human behaviour – and the thoughts, feelings, and motivations behind it – through observation, measurement, and testing, in order to form conclusions that are based on sound scientific methodology.

More than 100 years before, Watson (1913/1948), the famous behaviourist, defined psychology as:

> A purely objective experimental branch of natural science. Its theoretical goal is the prediction and control of behaviour. Introspection forms no essential part of its methods, nor is the scientific value of its data dependent upon the readiness with which they lend themselves to interpretation in terms of consciousness.

The tone of both these definitions is not that different. Words like 'observation', 'measurement', 'testing', 'sound scientific methodology', 'objective', 'prediction', and 'control' are the buzz words for post-positivist and logical empiricist outlooks on humans and their behaviour, not the words most would associate with words such as 'inclusion' and 'equality'. Does this indicate that psychology has gone around in a full circle or essentially remained linear from modern to contemporary psychology, but convinced itself that it has evolved with time because technology has changed and ideologies, norms, values, and communities have changed? Is contemporary/mainstream psychology fit for purpose in the 21st century? It seems harsh, but the powerbase within psychology in the UK lays within its membership based within divisions and faculties such as in clinical, forensic, educational, counselling, and health psychology at the British Psychological Society (see British Psychological Society, 2022). The dominant research base and practices of the people who are associated with these divisions are primarily quantitative, positivist, reductionist, and clinical (but not everyone) and therefore, there must be questions about how equality fits into that if those philosophical mindsets are in place. Compare that to the smaller 'Sections', which tend to be smaller groups of like-minded people interested in 'other' aspects of psychology within the British Psychological Society, they are not as powerful and influential in dictating how the discipline of psychology could be presented. Sections include interests in the political, community, women, sexualities, and qualitative methods – how would psychology look if these sections were the divisions? Could a new psychology emerge that might embrace the facets that a critical posthumanities perspective would present that would not put one psychology over another psychology? Dare we imagine psychology that is an assemblage, an uneven way of thinking about human behaviour and the mind to something that is still becoming?

That being said, mainstream psychology functions in a way that could relate to posthumanist thinking, depending on which angle you look at it. For example, the use of technology such as FaceGen, software that helps to generate faces or, EEG and TMS equipment, eye tracker systems, Oculus Rift, Cold Pressors, BioPac, and polygraph systems, all equipment that as allowed psychologists to explore how our minds and bodies work, and this for me fits with the transhumanist ideas of Bolstrom and Haraway's views on cyborgism (see Chapter 1). Psychologists have also used apps, social media, photovoice, and other digital and accessible equipment to engage with people and to find out about how their bodies, brains, and behaviour functions in day-to-day life. Some of this work has been done in collaboration with participants and many have found the use and engagement with the technologies mentioned empowering and life changing suggesting that there is some tacit acceptance for the need for relationality and blurring of divisions (see Reavey, 2021). Aside from the digital and scientific machines that have been used, many aspects of mainstream psychology have been driven by psychologists applying interventions within their work that are physical and mental health related, providing support and care for people in need, contributing to helping to save people's lives. This makes me think that for all the criticisms directed at what mainstream psychology represents, I am also lucky to be associated with excellent professionals who are motivated to make a difference in people's lives whether the differences applied are ameliorative or transformative. Now, I sound like a hypocrite because this sounds very different to the tone of this book so far. But, if I am suggesting that mainstream psychology is out-of-date and not as progressive as it thinks it is and needs to change, critics of psychology must also acknowledge that all psychologists have a contribution to make to help psychology move forward in a way that is inclusive and empowering for the people we work with in communities and alongside marginalised groups. Surely that tone would fit in with a critical posthumanities outlook on what psychology can become, moving beyond the established binaries and boundaries of what 'behaviour', 'mind', 'body', or 'human' that epitomises most psychology research and practice.

What is for sure is that the mainstream psychology that is in place and powerful will remain, for good or bad reasons. For instance, in the UK, higher education institutions must undergo a 'Research Excellence Framework' (REF) which is a process where institutions are assessed on the quality of their research. This dictates what level of funding an institute receives, and this is decided by expert panels in units of assessment, where outputs such as publications are assessed as well as the impact research has beyond academia and the environment that supports the research. For psychology, their unit of assessment comes under 'psychology, psychiatry and neuroscience', implying that psychology is intertwined with a strong medical and scientific discourse, and the latest edition of the REF reports that the UK continues to be a world leader in psychology, neuroscience, and psychiatry. This demonstrates the power of psychology and would suggest that it is unlikely to want to change if it is a world leader and receiving massive funds. For example, alongside neuroscience and psychiatry up to £2.7 billion pounds in external funding was awarded (2014–2020). The report that followed this process has indicated that psychological research has contributed towards reducing mortality, improving quality of life, and having impact on policy and legislation in all areas of day-to-day life and within major societal institutions at local, national, and international levels (Research Excellence Framework 2021, Overview Report by Main Panel A and Sub-Panels 1–6, 2022).

The report also states that new collaborations with stakeholders and international partners have been strengthened and that many of the outputs were rigorous and theory-led experimental research using both quantitative and qualitative methodologies. Yet, the core of the research outputs submitted was experimental research widely applied in developmental, educational, and occupational psychology. It does acknowledge however that qualitative approaches produced 'novel insights in diverse contexts' within health and public spaces, suggesting that not all the research was experimental and scientific. Furthermore, the report points out that there has been much improvement in work that has been done that promoted equality, diversity, and inclusion, with more engagement with race and disability groups and more emphasis on promoting BAME staff. On a positive note, then, there is more work being done with stakeholders beyond 'the lab' and international collaborations are continuing, and psychology is working across different disciplines, which implies that being completely critical and outspoken about mainstream psychology might be unfair. Then again, the principles, values, methods, and philosophical perspectives of psychologists, neuroscientists, and psychiatrists are rooted in reductionist and logical empiricist ways of 'doing psychology', and this brings in money, power and influence in ways that alienate marginalised groups and squeeze out more qualitative, creative, innovative methods that promote the voices of marginalised people and groups.

Despite this exclusion of marginalised people at the heart of psychological research, psychology as a discipline to study is very popular in the UK. Students and professionals recognise that they can develop transferable skills and build careers where they are motivated to help people and want to do good, even if to people like me the methods and practices are dated. But, whilst the skills and experiences help people to get better jobs and to build a career in psychology and beyond, it contributes to the unequal and damaging effects of neoliberal and capitalist societies, suggesting that psychology as a force is contributing to that by producing large quantities of graduates to use those skills and experiences to enhance those systems, but then again, we have to survive in that system and it cannot be a bad thing that people want to do well. How can I say that it is wrong when I have been through that journey and so have the biggest critics in psychology, who now live in nice homes, have luxury cars, travel the world, and have excellent pensions? The reality is that psychology is everywhere and within us and within our communities, so to be stuck on values of observation, experimentation, deduction, and value-free methods or be stuck on just being critical and not offering realistic alternatives, and essentially being an 'angry psychologist' alongside the 'ignorant psychologist', forms a binary that is unworkable and not in line with the progressive nature of our world.

The psychology that we know in the mainstream is not likely to change anytime soon. Nor will the stances of the critics of mainstream psychology. However, the contradiction of mainstream psychology is that it presents itself as a popular and powerful part of life and society, and arguably psychology is the fulcrum of how we understand humans in the 21st century. Yet, the very spine of mainstream psychology, practices, methods, and applications are primarily entrenched in old-fashioned ways of reductionism and empiricism that are alien approaches for marginalised people. A further complication here is that with psychology being so diverse, with so many psychologies, perspectives, and methods, psychology is also showing, but not admitting to being a good example of what a critical posthumanities psychology it really is and the potential it has for marginalised people. Psychology can be relational, plural, and uneven, but maybe the linear simplistic nature of psychology, and how it survives and remains powerful through neoliberal tendencies ensures that remains complicated and unsure of its identity in the context of marginalised people.

Summary

I began this chapter by thinking about one experience of when I explored 'intelligence' with a group of undergraduates' psychology students, in collaboration with a community group of people with disabilities. The vignette highlighted the problems with the simplification of what intelligence is or is not, and that intelligence is in fact complex, diverse, and connected to many things, not solely on how good you are at completing an IQ test, enshrined in logic, reason, mathematics and science. However, psychologists and mainstream psychology have explored this topic for a long time and the main understandings of how to view intelligence are still primarily encapsulated by logical empiricist and reductionist thinking.

This is no surprise when one explores the development of modern psychology. The build-up to Wundt and his psychology laboratory was dominated by a movement that turned from God and the soul to a movement that epitomised scientific ideas that are familiar in research and practice well into the 21st century, influenced in part by the West by British Associationalists and Mills's 'brick-wall hypothesis' alongside the development of psychophysics, physiognomy, and sensory psychophysiology. In other words, much of the forerunning ideas before Wundt's laboratory emerged were very much based on the assumption that there is a physiological basis for the minds that we have and develop. This means we can only be understood through scientific and experimental methods, through a process of observation and linear judgement, which is still at the heart of the UK's British Psychological Society's way of thinking about what psychology 'is'.

The rise of Wundt and the early behaviourists arguably set the tone for mainstream psychology as we know it today. Whilst behaviourist psychology is no longer the dominant paradigm within psychology, it still plays a part in the underpinning ideas that are connected to association learning that still influence clinical and educational practice, still leaving today's psychology with a clear link to a scientific and experimental past that you now see in different forms in neuropsychology and cyberpsychology. The simplicity of experiments and statistics, a reduction of who someone might be, rejects the possibilities of diversity and complex identities. Even the basics in Freud's theories and the psychodynamics thinkers that emerged thereafter, struggled to move beyond the problematic individual as opposed to problematic society and communities where people live. Yet, the ideas of Watson, Freud, Pavlov, and others live on and are very much manifested within the consciousness of mainstream psychology.

Despite the emergence of psychologies that have been 'humanistic', critical, or community orientated in nature, with strong qualitative and creative backdrops, and their influences on university programmes and research, the mainstream and contemporary psychology that we know remains underpinned by positivism, logical empiricism, and falsification. This ensures that ̶ ̶ ̶ ̶ ̶ ̶ ̶ ̶ ̶ psychology is mostly focused on reality being observed, ̶ ̶ ̶ ̶ ̶ ̶ d through scientific methods, that are value-free and ̶ ̶ ̶ ̶ al, political, social, and economic influences. The short ̶ ̶ ̶ of the UK and the Western development of psychology ̶ ̶ tream psychology is still in principle the same as it was a hundred years ago, despite the plethora of research, critiques, philosophies, and diverse methods that have emerged in the past 70 years.

Whilst I have suggested that on the whole that mainstream psychology has not changed, I do think all psychologies have something to offer on how we might understand 'humans' and their contexts and how we intersect with the world around us. The epicentre of what mainstream psychology is, is also accompanied by the emergence of different perspectives and different methods, and society and people have changed over these decades too, so actually psychology is in a good place to emerge as a psychology that is becoming that can really be relational across societies, communities, people, and beyond. There is hope and opportunity for change, if psychologists really want to change, changes that could develop psychology into something that is inclusive and that can work as equals with marginalised people. This makes me think about Goodley's idea in relation to critical disability studies in that we may start with disabilities, but not end with disabilities because all that encompasses our understanding of disabilities through the political, theoretical, practices, and labelling of disability is relevant to everyone (see Goodley, 2011, 2013). In a similar way, we need to think about 'psychology' and what it means and its influences, power, practices, identities, and applications before we can seek to find new ways of thinking and visioning what 'psychology' can become in such a way that we do not end or continue with the psychology that we have come to know.

Arguably, aspects of this have already taken place in psychology with the emergence of different psychologies over the past 70 years and even in the past 20 years as can be seen within organisations like the British Psychological Society in the UK such as cyberpsychology, political psychology, women, and men's psychology (British Psychological Society, 2022). One other psychology that is less spoken about, but as a concept has arguably been around for 60 plus years is 'community psychology'. As I stated earlier in this book, being introduced to critical community psychology was a revelation that gave me hope about what psychology could become beyond the reductionist principles that underpin mainstream psychology. This will be explored further in the next chapter with a view to thinking about what it is has done and could do to influence change and how it might link with a critical posthumanities perspective.

3 Community psychology – Mainstream psychology or hope for what psychology can become?

Chapter 2 presented a brief and vague overview of how contemporary psychology has developed and what it represents in the 21st century, at least from my perspective. I have no doubt that psychologists are professional, focused on making a difference, and are dedicated to seeing psychology progress; however, the established philosophical position for many psychologists and mainstream psychologists is forged in logical empiricist and reductionist thinking that can be seen through its application, practices, and methods. This raises questions on whether mainstream psychology is fit for purpose way into the 21st century. Yes, I often reflect on the 'elephant in the room' and regularly reflect on this with my students and colleagues about why with all my qualifications, interests, and successes in the name of 'psychology', I spend a lot of time challenging what it means and why I think it is flawed. I think there are two reasons why I continue to remain connected to psychology. First, it helps me maintain and get jobs because 'psychology' can be used in many organisations, associations, and establishments because of the skills and experiences you develop in practice or from research meaning my skills are transferable and useful, but ultimately, it helps to pay the mortgage and gives me stability in life within the neoliberal and capitalist systems in which we all live in. Secondly, it cannot be doubted that I am passionate about psychology and its potential to make a difference in people's lives. Yes, I do think all-round that contemporary psychology and its current state is essentially entrenched within dated reductionist philosophies and methodologies, but I also think that it is powerful and influential enough to change the world so that people can live in a value-based context that seeks to promote the voices of marginalised people. I live in hope and hope that I will continue to live in hope going forward that psychology can be a becoming psychology and I will scribble down some reflections later in the book about what this might mean under a 'posthuman community psychology'.

The way I have presented psychology in Chapter 2 would suggest that my hopes for psychology to be more value-based and to promote the voices of marginalised people is very unlikely whilst mainstream psychology remains the same. Psychology is powerful and driven by the same values that underpin medical models of mental health and by multi-billion-pound

DOI: 10.4324/9781003057673-3

drug industries alongside powerful technology and influences (see Condie & Richards, 2022), and therefore, to imagine a psychology that is always in flux is complicated, especially when in other ways, like humans, it changes too. Yet, the thinkers, writers, and practitioners that emerged in the 1960s to lay the foundations for a critical psychology, challenging the status quo that permeates through Western psychology and beyond, provided some hope and we can see that in how qualitative research and methodologies are now common in the teaching of psychology and has been for decades. Albeit in small amounts, we can also see through the development of less mainstream psychologies such as those based at the British Psychological Society in the UK that an all-encompassing scientific and psychologising psychology alone is not possible, so there is some hope that mainstream psychology can adapt and be flexible to new ideas and perspectives that might reach out to all people in many ways, genuinely promoting values relating to diversity, inclusion, and equality.

In my introduction to the book, I referred to my frustrations with psychology and acknowledged that a moment in time provided me with a new insight and positivity about what psychology could be beyond the laboratory. When I was introduced to 'community psychology', I felt that there was then some hope that psychology could be a force for change and difference in a way that I had not seen in psychology regardless of the past 50 years of critique and the outcomes from the so called 'crisis in social psychology'. In fact, it was around the time of the 'crisis' that arguably 'community psychology' emerged to challenge the stoic and scientific psychology that had been established. With this in mind, this chapter explores some of the meanings behind 'community psychology' and its place within and around psychology, at least in the first instance, from my perspective. The chapter is not aiming to cover all types and meanings of 'community psychology' because there are many simple and complicated perspectives on what it is. But the chapter will allude to what community psychology means to most, and its place going forward, and some reflections on two streams of community psychology that will be briefly explored interchangeably, that being 'mainstream' and 'critical' community psychology. The chapter will provide a critical taste to community psychology's possibilities and its problems, which will be explored further in Chapter 4 where I discuss community psychology 'in action' with marginalised groups using my experiences and reflections, in line with the queerying nature of this book.

This chapter focuses on my understanding of what critical/community psychology is to me and what has driven my practice and teaching of critical/community psychology. Therefore, there will be a focus on not just acknowledging the difficulties in defining community psychology and the tensions between mainstream and critical community psychologists at an international level, but on specific principles that have meant something to me or have been at the heart of my work. For example, in terms of thinking about people in context, social justice, the voices of 'other', visual, creative, and digital methods, decolonialisation and deideologisation, sharing expertise and participation and the significance of inter/intra/interdisciplinary work. These areas of thinking in relation to community psychology encompass much of what most versions of community psychology promote in different contexts, and mine on an individual level.

To give a taste of what a community psychology approach might look like, from my interpretation and application of a critical/community psychology approach, the vignette is one piece of work I helped to facilitate and create, and before I reflect on critical/community psychology in more detail, maybe this is a moment for you to reflect on why this is different to the mainstream psychology that we know and think about, but why it is still 'psychology' or whether is it an example of critical or mainstream community psychology (see Richards (2022) for another version of the vignette below).

Critical/Community 'psychology' in action!

'Our Advocacy' was a self-advocacy group, which aimed to set up partnerships between volunteers and adults with intellectual disabilities of different genders, ethnicities, and sexualities, over the age of 18. By building up a relationship between the volunteer and member of the project, the members could access the community more and take part in activities, achieving a stronger likelihood of inclusion and full participation, with their voices at the heart of the project.

The development of Our Advocacy emerged when some members of the advocacy project had expressed that they wanted to meet more people, and they wanted to take part in more activities. An idea materialised from one of the members of the group that it might be more productive if volunteers learned more about the lives of people with intellectual disabilities through the sharing of experiences through drama, art, poetry, and dialogue. Therefore, the group wanted to deliver a type of training that involved sharing experiences and knowledge about living with intellectual disabilities to promote their voices relating to issues to do with the control of money, sexuality, sex and relationships, and bullying.

For example, the aim of the drama scenes was to engage volunteers, to help them become more aware of how people with intellectual disabilities are treated and how they wanted to be treated. Once the drama scenes were completed, the group and volunteers would discuss what took place, with the aim to help the volunteers to think more about the issues people with intellectual disabilities face daily.

Most volunteers who took part said it helped them to think more about what it was like to have intellectual disabilities, and this would help them to judge people with intellectual disabilities differently in the future. Other volunteers were confused about what the drama scenes concerned and how it related to them, but were willing to learn more to understand more, and they felt that this was important in their role as a volunteer.

3 hours later ....

Calon, one of the members of the project, was collected by a special local bus service, that was especially ordered so that he could get home safely. The people on the bus were known to him because he would see them regularly at the end of activities from places he was taken. They too had intellectual disabilities and they were not allowed to get on a public bus on their own. When Calon left the bus, he was greeted by his sister, his live-in carer, and his coat was taken off him and he was taken to the dining room where he would eat his dinner silently whilst watching a small television. Once he ate the last chip on his plate, it was time for Calon to get ready for bed, at about 7 pm. He was told that he must feel tired and that there was not much on television to watch. He walked upstairs to the bathroom where his clothes that his carer had chosen were ready and he took a shower. He was asked constantly through the door if he was ok, and like he did every other night of the week, he told her that he was ok. When he dried himself and brushed his teeth, he walked to his room and got into bed, with the usual 'goodnight and God bless' being exchanged between him and his carer. Calon would sometimes go straight to sleep, but most of the time, he sat thinking through the predictable routines that would take place at breakfast, dinner, and supper, and he would know exactly which shops, activities, and people he would be experiencing because that is what he would do week in and week out. How would he ever find a partner? How would he ever have privacy and be able to make choices? Who would ever know who he really was? Where was Calon's voice?

What is 'community psychology' to me?

Before presenting the vignette that provided some insight into one example of what a critical/community psychology project or approach might look like, I proposed thinking about how this is different to mainstream psychology and whether it is psychology or is it mainstream or critical community psychology (more to come on this later). The example suggests that it is different to mainstream psychology because the project and actions that took place were within a local community and not in a controlled environment. It is different because a marginalised group of people worked together to develop the project, ensuring that to some extent, it was a bottom-up approach, where decisions, ideas, and actions were agreed, and the activities appear to have been driven by the 'participants' rather than just the 'facilitators', implying that it was inclusive. The project provided a platform for the group to promote their voices and to think and act in a way that was creative and empowering. So, just in those couple of sentences alone, there is already a sense that this was a different type of psychology in action, different from the mainstream psychology and top-down approaches that rely on traditional forms of method and analysis such as experiments, structured surveys, interviews, and questionnaires, with clear quantitative analyses. For me, this resonates with a 'critical community psychology' approach to action that focuses on oppression and liberation, critical constructionism, a focus on challenging systems that are unjust and there was solidarity with workers and members of that community through a critical praxis (Fox et al., 2009). There were aspects of participatory action research, wellbeing, and collaboration, that may be different to what might be labelled as 'mainstream community psychology' that some have related to individual competence and a post-positivist perspective, albeit mainstream community psychology emerged as a protest against mainstream psychology, concerned with social justice and social action (Evans et al., 2017. But the vignette acknowledged that whilst a different type of psychology is being described, the project and activities and for all its work in promoting inclusivity, the project was ameliorative in nature and did not transform the lives of the people who participated. Therefore, it is also important to note that from the outset of this chapter, I am conscious that for all the positive views of community psychology that I lean towards and my negative narratives about mainstream psychology, both have flaws and complications that ensure that the voices of marginalised people are limited, ensuring that transformative change in people's lives is very difficult.

For some, the vignette would not be considered 'psychology' at all because this kind of work would be alien to many psychologists. However, as discussed in Chapter 2, over the past 70 years, many have written that psychology is not and should not be just about the laboratory but should be a psychology that is for the people in that people should be judged in context, by people who are value-driven and want to work with people and not on people. That being said, even with the onset of inclusive qualitative methods and methodologies being incorporated into psychology curriculums, and in recent years in particular (see Reavey, 2021), the onset of visual methods and digital technology that have been useful tools to engage with communities within psychology, but psychology has still struggled to connect with marginalised people. My critical and cynical analysis of the discipline of psychology in Chapter 2 highlighted these issues, and even when I highlighted the positives or the opportunities, I still come back to the question, 'does psychology promote the voices of marginalised people in society?'. When most people think about psychology, they think about very traditional notions of psychology. People might think about therapists and clinicians, or people might think about treatment of mental health problems or how people think, perceive, or behave, or one-to-one interventions, or the many documentaries or television shows that reinforce and true and not-so-true stereotypes of what psychologists are. What is for sure is that these examples reflect a medicalised and pathologised view of psychology, and those views are not just partly stereotypical, but a genuine reality for many people.

These psychologising perspectives in tone are all about fixing and prescribing or 'sorting someone out'. For me, this was never what psychology should be or could be about. I have described myself as a critical community psychologist and this seemed the right thing to do because for me, this was the only psychology, along with psychologies such as liberation and peace psychology, with influences from queer theory, critical social theory and poststructuralism, that I felt connected too. For me, this really helped to capture and encompass a value-laden, contextualised psychology that promotes voicing social justice, climate change, participatory action research and is prepared to work across disciplines to build allies and be open to visual and creative methods in a way that mainstream psychology as never been. Therefore, community psychology, in whatever form, is a psychology that gives me hope that mainstream psychology can move forward in a way that allows psychology to become a psychology for marginalised people in society. This hope is enhanced further for me when I think of what a critical posthumanities underpinning could be and how the ideas could infiltrate psychology to help psychology to review itself as something that is ambiguous and uneven, like the people they study. Anyway, that is me, so what has community psychology become?

What has 'community psychology' become?

So, you're a clinical psychologist?

Over the years, I have spent a lot of time giving talks, presentations, delivering lectures, and having general chats with people about what I do and what I have done. I generally say that I am a critical community psychologist, acknowledging that my influences have primarily come from the work of critical community psychologists who were based at Manchester Metropolitan University in the past. I will generally relay to people what critical community psychologists believe, compared to mainstream psychology, such as a belief in seeing people in context, social justice issues, being value-laden, community action, prevent problems rather than fix problems, and so on. In the same conversations, I might then provide some examples of my own work or the other work of other critical/community psychologists relating to issues to do with climate change, homelessness, poverty, gender rights, and men's health, amongst others. I sometimes show pictures of my work or the work of others and advise on links to websites that might provide more information and insight into critical/community psychology.

I have done the above many times, and many times, the response back has been, 'so are you a clinical psychologist?'. This has led to me being presented as a clinical psychologist at presentations, events, and discussions. Maybe it is the way I say things or maybe it is because it is difficult for people, within psychology and beyond, to comprehend a psychology that is different to mainstream psychology. Similarly, community psychologists and I have experienced comments such as, 'so what is community psychology'? 'Is it clinical psychology?', 'It sounds like sociology … are you sure you are not a sociologist?' This tells me that in general people do not know what critical/community psychology is or have never heard of it. I would suggest then that considering the concept has been around for nearly 60 years, it has always had an identity crisis, like mainstream psychology, and that can be seen in its many definitions, methodologies, and interpretations, probably in a way that mainstream psychology has never faced, and maybe in part why mainstream psychology continues to have the status quo on what people view psychology as being.

The reflection about the meaning of 'critical/community psychology' from the perspective of people that I have met suggests that for all my narratives of what critical/community psychology means to me and what I think it is, I find in general that people cannot comprehend a psychology that is beyond the laboratory, or a prison or hospital or counselling room. For most people, I come across when I speak about critical/community psychology, I get an eyebrow raised, or a 'well done' for sounding 'left wing' and being nice about speaking up for marginalised groups or a look of fear if I sound too radical. This might highlight that critical/community psychology is not just difficult to define and comprehend away from the mainstream, but maybe like mainstream psychology, it has an identity crisis. For example, even within critical/community psychology, there are differences of opinion about the meaning, definitions, applications, and methods of what a community psychologist is. Whilst the common and established founding of community psychology is said to have taken place in 1965 at the Swampscott conference, others will say that it began much earlier (Fryer, 2008). Some would say that critical/community psychology has been critical from the outset, because of the challenges it makes against mainstream psychology, whereas others will say that mainstream community psychology is not a lot different to mainstream psychology, with words like 'community', 'social justice', and 'inclusion' stamped on work for political reasons (Evans et al., 2017).

The mainstream community psychology that emerged in the 1960s, the 'USA version', stemmed in part from the emergence of humanistic psychology and the influences of the civil rights movements of the 1950s and 1960s, as noted in Chapter 2, and helped to dent the entrenched reductionist standing of the discipline of psychology. In addition to this, frustrations were emerging about the medical model of mental health, which generally benefits the middle classes and above and the lack of recognition of the importance of people in context. There was frustration that psychologists were ignoring or not considering in their work the societal issues their clients faced. The conversations that took place at Swampscott, influenced strongly by clinical psychologists, emphasised the need for more representation from marginalised groups within psychology with more focus on prevention than treating the individual and seeking change to systems (see Tebes, 2016). The conference emerged to outline what a 'community mental health' approach could mean, with conversations around psychologists becoming active participants in research and practice, and more emphasis on prevention and evaluation through research and working with people rather than on them (Bennet et al., 1966; Rickel, 1987). Within this, you could say that prevention, social justice, and an ecological understanding for people were directly emerging within psychology in a way like never before, albeit that people within psychology long before the 1960s were talking about some of these values, but maybe not as comprehensively in the mainstream.

Whilst some critical community psychologists would dispute the extent mainstream community psychology has been critical and political, at least conversations about what psychology should be or what it could become were starting to be discussed more and more. Some writers that have discussed the emergence and continuation of community psychology on a global front (see Reich & Reich, 2006; Vazquez Rivera, 2010), with lots of similarities in terms of the overall goals already mentioned, and authors such as Fryer and Laing (2008) and Gridley and Breen (2007), have highlighted that community psychology itself is contested in relation to geography and time and contexts (also see Kagan et al., 2021). Therefore, community psychology is continuing to evolve, meaning that it is difficult to say what community psychology is and what it can become, which is maybe a better way to think about psychology. This has all been the more possible with the emergence of political and radical perspectives that are associated with community psychology in all its varieties. What is for sure is that whatever 'community psychology' is, it is something that resonates with psychologists and their allies in many places, even if not at the same scale as interest in mainstream psychology. Reich et al.'s (2007) work is a useful example of community psychology's outreach and diversity across the world, with a collection of varied and worldly examples of the beginnings and values of community psychologists from different countries that are not just entrenched, as is often the case, within European-American-Western settings.

Although mainstream community psychology can be challenged for its associations with the mainstream psychology that it is meant to challenge in the first place. The 'critical' has emerged in different places within community psychology influenced by 'critical community psychologists', who have arguably taken the challenge further by reflecting on how far mainstream community psychology has come and what it could do better. For example, you can see this with some USA-based community psychologists who have started to apply more critical perspectives in recent times into their work where they highlight the importance of the political and liberation and seek more radical solutions to entrenched societal problems (Nelson & Prilleltensky, 2005). Also, the authors based and connected to the UK have provided ideas and perspectives that are 'critical' and have promoted the need for criticality in practice and research over recent decades (see Kagan et al., 2021), if at not least for the need to critically rethink what 'community' means (Coimbra et al., 2012) and to think critically about place and function of power (see Sloan, 1996; Fisher et al., 2007). For me, this version of community psychology was what got me hooked into how I thought that psychology could actually change the world and make a difference. From my own personal experiences of poverty, abuse, marginalisation, and exclusion and from witnessing that with other people and groups in society, the political and radical nature of this part of psychology was refreshing. This was a psychology that compared to mainstream psychology and mainstream community psychology made me more aware of the influences of power over maintaining social injustice and how capitalism, colonialisation, patriarchy, and neoliberal globalisation manifested itself into communities. The ideas of working with people, taking social action, and building relationships and making allies with our community partners were exciting and liberating. But why critical community psychology and not mainstream community psychology?

I have already alluded to some differences, but Fox et al. (2009) provided some useful ideas about the differences between mainstream and critical community psychology. For example, mainstream is less political and focused on individual competence. Critical community psychology focuses more on oppression and liberation and solidarity between professionals and community members through praxis (see Evans et al., 2017). Indeed, there are crossovers relating to ecology, value-laden, aspects of participatory action research, wellbeing, and collaboration. All-in-all, some clear binaries between both streaks of community psychology, and some overlaps too. Is this really a surprise? The development of community psychology from Swampscott was driven by clinical psychologists, albeit with a passion for social action and change, but nevertheless, trained, influenced, and practised like the mainstream psychologists that they were, and many continue to be, ensuring that a critical, liberal and heterogeneous approaches and practices to psychology will be limited, and easy for it to be picked at by critics. For example, has mainstream community psychology really been about having a 'special interest' in social justice issues, but when it comes to radical change, has not even touched the surface? Maybe so, and this would not be a shock with the limited philosophies, theories and new ideas, radical ideas that have emerged in other disciplines but not in this one, shoehorning out anything that is too political. It seems to me that whatever version of community psychology you consider, the values that all sides of community psychology profess to being at the heart of their practices and research do not have transformative effects, and arguably, maintain a similar position as mainstream psychology, just using different words or words that sound good like 'inclusion', 'empowerment', and 'participation'.

There has been much criticism for 'USA-based' community psychology that is often seen as the flag bearer for 'mainstream community psychology', yet the historical setup in the UK has been similar and can still be seen today. For instance, it was clinical psychologists that dominated the Swampscott conference, and it was those psychologists that were angry about what psychology was about and what it had become. Similarly, Burton et al. (2007) point out that it was the work of Bender and Tully, clinical psychologists, that started to put 'community psychology' as a concept on the map in the UK and Bender's (1976) book was really the first to introduce community psychology in the UK context, meaning that like USA community psychology, UK community psychology has emerged from frustrated clinical psychologists (also see Dutta, 2018). Whilst Burton et al. (2007) suggested that community psychology emerged in waves rather than a definitive point in time like Swampscott, the term 'community psychology' was not really used until Swampscott and in the UK, community psychology had been slow in being seen as a movement that challenges the power of psychology. For example, that slowness continues today, even with the development of a 'Community Psychology Section' within the British Psychological Society UK, in 2010. Despite the energy and enthusiasm to challenge mainstream psychology, Festivals of Community Psychology (Hadjiosif & Desai, 2022) and various activities and action that has taken place to promote community psychology, broadly speaking, there have been no changes made in how people view psychology, and mainstream psychology has not been affected or changed in any way. If anything, the Section's collusion with mainstream psychology has allowed mainstream psychology to gobble up another psychology for its collection (and I am an inside witness to this Section). An additional problem within the UK context that is often ignored is the division between mainstream community psychologists and critical community psychologists, and this can arguably be seen within a geographical north-south divide. There is lots of talk from mainstream community psychologists about 'inclusion', 'empowerment' or 'let's change psychology', but any sniff of real radical change from the critical community psychologists, and any chance for real change or a real challenge to mainstream psychology is shied away from. There are regular patterns of 'stamping of feet' for social justice issues in conversations about community psychology in the UK context, but doing this directly in collaboration, with a view to facilitate bottom-up approaches with marginalised people, is rare. This means that the voices of mainstream/critical community psychologists in the UK who are mostly made up of people with the same identities that mainstream psychology is criticised for being – white, middle-class, wealthy, and educated (like me), continue to prevail above the voices of marginalised people. It seems to me that critical/community psychology is used to vent some frustrations from time to time about a social justice issue, but that is far as it ever really goes, making critical/community psychology a 'special issue' psychology rather than one that could transform mainstream psychology and the lives of marginalised people. Maybe mainstream community psychology has stayed like mainstream psychology because without that, it would not be taken as seriously by mainstream psychologists. Maybe in the UK, if community psychology became too radical, would the British Psychological Society want the Section to remain? Do we need to straddle between what we challenge and what we are prepared to accept and conform to, for any chance for change to happen? Whatever way you look at it, it is difficult to see how critical/community psychology in any established form can fulfil its goals of change, liberation, and accompaniment whilst the psychologising of psychology continues, and whilst there remains a binary between mainstream and critical community psychologies replicating the similar binary between mainstream and critical psychology in the UK.

It seems bizarre that for a discipline that is focused on collaboration, solidarity, and eagerness for change that there seems to be more division, and those divisions are not spoken about enough and part of this is because how community psychologists interpret community psychology and how they define it and 'do' it, which is problematic. In terms of defining 'community psychology', critical or mainstream, the academic way, it has been primarily defined from a Western, Eurocentric perspective, despite the strong influences and connections across all areas of the world. This adds more complexity and diversity to what community psychology means, suggesting community psychology is always emerging, becoming, and not fixed, but it is worth reflecting on some keywords and tenets that have traditionally been set out about what it means, with these words specifically associated with Swampscott (Rappaport, 1977; Dalton et al., 2001; Fryer & Laing, 2008; Kagan et al., 2011, 2021):

1   Individual vs. system change.
2   Action.
3   Empowerment and social justice.
4   Strengths, resilience, prevention, and promotion.
5   Diversity and context.
6   Collaboration.

If you add other words and perspectives to this, including liberation, solidarity, accompaniment, deideologisation, critical consciousness, words associated with a more critical community psychology outlook, you have an all-encompassing community psychology that can be a community for all, which links with a critical posthumanities perspective that I presented in Chapter 1. Regardless of whether you position yourself as a mainstream or critical community psychologist, the words from Swampscott and wordings from others later, were and are extraordinary in the context of psychology, and if actioned, equally as powerful now in word and practice, psychology and the world would be a different place. It might be useful, therefore, to think about the commonalities between all of us and how we think and feel about what psychology and people should be about is more similar than what psychologists like to admit to.

Another way to think about community psychology is to note that much work has been done that feels like mainstream/critical community psychology but is 'placed' elsewhere whilst having similar values and methods, such as youth work (Kagan et al., 2021; also see Lawthom et al., 2007). The main ideas that stand out and make community psychology different, whether mainstream or critical, is the importance of going beyond the individualistic perspective and instead placing emphasis on the surrounding contexts. One of the tenets that sets out community psychology to be different, when compared to other forms of psychology, is that of it being value-based, even if there are arguments for whether it is laden or driven by values, like the ideas referred to in the introduction chapter of the book of justice, stewardship, and community (Kagan et al., 2021). This form of critical/community psychology overlaps with other forms of community psychology in other parts of the world, and within aspects of mainstream community psychology, and attempts to depart from traditional approaches in psychology in that it places problems and issues individuals, groups, and communities face, in their contexts and not within the individual (see Nelson & Prilleltensky, 2005). The concept of the 'ecological metaphor' considers the different environments that we may encounter during our lifespan, that can influence behaviour at different times and situations. In relation to this, what sets critical community psychology apart (and other forms of community psychology) from an 'individualised' psychology is the way critical/community psychologists seek explanations of social experience and taking action (Kagan et al., 2011). Therefore, applying an ecological perspective has become an important principle of critical/community psychology theory and practice, considering a person/people within the contexts that surround them, which enables critical and mainstream community psychologists to develop new progressive insights (Kloos et al., 2021).

From my perspective, what epitomises community psychology to me, whether I jump from being a critical or mainstream community psychologist, or straddle between these fuzzy binaries, is going beyond the individual and seeing people in context. With a view not to focus problems of life on a person and to try and 'fix' them, but to recognise them as complex identities in a complex world that needs to change to help and care for people. In addition, for me, social justice needs to be at the heart of any form of community psychology whether that be protesting for gender rights or supporting trans people whatever age, or climate change, or helping the homeless or people who are facing mental health difficulties, these and many more social justice issues should be at the very heart of all forms of psychology. To be able to do this, I have always felt that the voices of marginalised people need to be promoted through bottom-up approaches using methods that are accessible, engaging, creative and fun, and for it to be a psychology with multi-disciplinary psychologists that are relational and likely to really help the marginalised to feel more empowered and included. I recognise this more when I think back to my childhood and even more so when I think back to working with marginalised people facing exclusionary practices in day-to-day life. This view may serve a way in which to challenge the structured economic powerbases that prop up mainstream psychology, but where mainstream psychology can be useful through the expertise and skills that mainstream psychologists can offer, then we should work with them. The decolonising and deideologising psychology would strengthen this further to become a psychology for the people, and for me, what community psychology aims to do helps to make all this possible to challenge the conservative and powerfully established ways of mainstream psychology. With these feelings in mind, I will now provide some further reflections into some of these areas and what community psychologists have done to promote some of these ideals. These sections represent what I think has been a core part of my work, but these values/principles are likely to be at the heart of many other community psychologists too, mainstream, or critical.

Going beyond the gaze of the individual – Ecology, community, and Other

Much has been discussed within community psychology about 'ecology theory' or the 'ecological metaphor' (Kelly, 1968; Kagan et al., 2021), and this generally concerns how people adapt in their contexts and how people have to work together to make use of resources to survive and prosper. This is useful for community psychologists of all kinds and the professionals and community members they work with because by understanding how the context of their world is made up, then you can begin to identify the social issues that people face. Moreover, to think about this also means that critical/community psychologists are likely to be interested in systems and to consider the systems at different levels of analysis, and by doing so, you are understanding the person in context rather than just focusing on the individual level of analysis, which is very much what mainstream psychology concerns.

Kelly's (1968) theory (and future developments of the theory by people such as Trickett, 2009) is still useful for critical/community psychologists

today and differs from mainstream psychology. The theory helps to understand the ways people interact and relate to one another and a stronger perspective can emerge on how best to help people and work with people to
develop interventions. Through adapting to change and recognising the
interconnective nature of communities, the sharing of resources and development of networks where expertise, skills and relationships are built, people
can support one another, through emotional or physical support and thus
resonates with a symbiotic and interconnected critical posthumanities outlook. Importantly, a core principle in this theory, and through many people's
definitions of critical/community psychology is the acknowledgement for
change and that communities and people are always changing, meaning that
adapting and evolving is a crucial part of communities and life. This may
also contribute to the level of what a sense of community might mean to
people and their communities too. How connected people feel might determine how change works and how networks form and promote the sharing
of resources. From a critical/community psychology perspective, the goal is
different to mainstream psychology is that the aim was to use research and
action at a community level, thus contributing positively to the local good
and contributing knowledge to research (see Bennet et al., 1966). By doing
so, an examination can be made of the complex systems and interconnections
between people and communities, with a view to collaborating and having
a shared understanding of the roles and norms and relationships within the
contexts that people live in. These ideas fit well with critical posthumanity
ideas relating to companionship and mutuality and highlight that the individual level of focus that dominates psychology is an old-fashioned way to
view ever-changing people and communities.

For all types of critical/community psychologist, an ecological perspective in some form on how we view people and communities is still
important because it can help form the basis of intervention and potential
transformative change for the social good, whilst incorporating cultural,
social, political, historical norms, and influences that contribute to the
identities of people and their communities. This may go some way into
understanding communities and marginalised groups, or Other', because
by understanding systems and the ecological makeup of a community, it is
more likely that you can gain insights into the prejudices, discriminations
and labelling that attaches itself to excluded groups (Richards et al., 2018).
Indeed, a primary goal for critical/community psychologists is to promote
the voices of the most marginalised and this can be linked with a sense of
community. Prilleltensky (2019) discussed the 'psychology of mattering'
where it can be said that people need to feel valued and add value too, this in
turn can make a difference in the lives of people and people that they know
and can be linked to classic buzz words in critical/community psychology
such as empowerment, respect, equality, and self-determination. However,
'Other' fits in with powerful neoliberal ideologies which dominate the West,
which makes sure there will remain the privileged few over the many, a

powerbase that is rhizomatic and strongly above community and wellbeing. This prioritises personal responsibility and freedoms, entrepreneurship, and individuality that contributes towards communities and the core values of critical/community psychology being blockaded by entrenched capitalism. These premises of an overpowering capitalist and neoliberal systems ensure that the most marginalised remain that way. For critical/community psychologists and their core values to prosper, the 'Other' needs to be central to practice, applications, methods, and ideologies that make up the diverse nature of critical/community psychology.

Social Justice – Empowerment and equalities

The real turn away from mainstream psychology for most critical/community psychologists was the focus on social justice issues. Therefore, for the most part, critical/community psychologists are interested in the ways in which social justice issues can be prevented and how they can be tackled, so issues relating to oppression, exclusion, and exploitation are important areas of concern. Examples of social justice issues are vast, but often relate to individual issues to do with race, marginalised sexualities, poverty, or wider, organisational, and societal issues to do with health inequalities and discriminatory practices within organisations. Recent work around social justice issues includes building alliances with local communities for people who face complicated housing systems (Carey et al., 2022), overcoming mental distress and marginalisation through community supported agriculture (Zoli et al., 2022), psychologists taking action for LGBT+ groups and their rights and wellbeing in the Philippines (Manalastas et al., 2022), the use of community arts in the context of decolonisation and Aboriginal self-determination (Quayle & Sonn, 2019; Sonn et al., 2022b) and building partnerships for community based service learning in poverty-stricken communities (Akhurst & Msomi, 2022). Of course, the list goes on in many contexts where community projects and research papers will talk about 'social justice' in all its complexities with elements of activism, with much written and analysed from a theoretical perspective. But social justice movements that have action and activism at their heart have also developed. For example, in the UK, the 'psychologists for social change' activist network has emerged as a series of different groups and structures that have social and political action as their core value, influenced by established UK and international thinkers of community psychology including Freire (1970), Smail (1994), and Martin-Baro (1994) and survivor and social justice movements (see Walker et al., 2022). They have sought to mobilise psychologists who are angry and frustrated with what marginalised people face by thinking of psychological work as political. Their call for action boasts values that are sometimes seen in critical/community psychology, but seldom seen in mainstream psychology, when social justice issues should be the primary focus of all psychologists, including values relating to being brave, visionary, being collective, taking action, be reflective, connecting, and having solidarity. These values can also be seen in protests and movements such as the MeToo campaign and Black Lives Matter (2018–2022).

Whilst there are places in the world that have produced laws to protect people facing issues to do with social justice such as race and gender equalities, other places do not have that protection, and some claim to promote equal opportunities for all, but it never quite happens for most. Social justice, therefore, is concerned not just with the feelings and emotions of one person and what they experience in context, but it is to do with distribution of resources, mutuality between people and greater access to support, even when there are differences in beliefs, values, and ideologies. For a critical/community psychologist or any other psychologist, social justices are central to their work because it encapsulates the very identities of all of us who live within the communities that we do. To share resources, build relationships and make way for better access for marginalised people benefits us all and this encapsulates ideas around mutuality from a critical posthumanities viewpoint. But specific groups continuously do not have the opportunity to experience this, and so for any form of psychology to claim that diversity and inclusivity are important to them, rather than just being 'feel good words' of the day, then we are all responsible for social justice issues, that are actually at the core of all our lives. Other forms of psychology that have a similar flavour to the value-led orientation of critical/community psychology and social justice issues, include liberation and peace psychology, and Martin-Baro (1994) noted that this kind of psychology is about what needs to be done rather than celebrating what has been done, and in this way, there is more of an opportunity to transform the world for the better rather than just trying to understand it.

Tools and methods – Promoting the voices of 'Other' through creativity

Thinking about people in context and social justice are key values for most critical/community psychologists, who are keen to take some form of action to make a difference, at a micro or macro level, but this means that tools and methods are needed to move away from experiments, observational behaviour, quantitative analysis, and other scientific forms of data collection and analysis. For example, critical/community psychology is most associated with and has a rich history in the use of participatory action research and other participatory methods, alongside mixed and multiple methods that encompass both qualitative and quantitative methods (Kagan et al., 2021). Participatory action research concerns knowledge sharing and action in collaboration with community members as a form of 'conscientisation', an important tenet that emphasises the need for awareness-raising and 'deindoctrination' with to address inequalities, within the philosophies of Paulo Freire (Freire, 1970; Reason, 1994; Reason & Bradbury, 2001). This form of research promotes the need for co-working with co-researchers in the community, a more equal partnership between psychologist and community members, working together to define problems and share information and take action, whilst reflecting together on this process. Participatory action research is in line with the core values of many critical/community psychologists such as empowerment and equality, flat-lining power where possible.

The use of a variety of tools and methods beyond the established tools and methods that are familiar to psychologists fits in with the bottom-up approaches and participatory work critical/community psychologists aim to do with community members and marginalised people. Community psychological methods usually relate to the development of ethnographies and are phenomenological in nature, but it has moved with the times in part too. With focus on experiences and voices of participants or co-collaborators, and the data or voices from these approaches still tending to still relate to traditional qualitative methods like interviews and focus groups, the use of technology through Photovoice, apps, social media and online networks have also become part of the process of working with community participants, albeit more is needed (Stein et al., 2019).

Interdisciplinary – Intersectional and multi-disciplinary psychology

In Chapter 2, my narrative was framed around that psychology reinforces the medical, and experimental models that engulf mainstream psychological practices. Yet, if a critical/community psychology or other rebellious forms of psychology concern social issues that are complex, messy, and intertwined, acknowledged through an ecological, contextual perspective, then there must be collaboration and connections with different disciplines and professionals to provide a more holistic understanding of the issues that marginalised people face. For example, in my own work, I know I have cut across different disciplines such as sociology, community development, social work, disability studies, philosophy as well as worked with the professionals within those areas. How could I not if trying to understand social issues and to find the best ways to prevent issues? This also is in line with values of empowerment and relationship building where people can gain from one another and contribute to a collective collaboration.

In academia, there is an obsession in recent years that research will be more highly regarded and have more kudos if mixed methods are used, but how highly regarded are t-tests for marginalised people? Why would people who are trying to survive each day be interested in creative, qualitative, or quantitative methods or analyses in research? However, more researchers from different disciplines are recognising that cross-collaboration within and between different disciplines and backgrounds can bring different knowledge and introduce new methods and increase the qualities of our practices and reflections on how we facilitate work, so in the same way that our skills might be transferable, other aspects of our work can be transferable. I referred to the Research Excellence Framework in the UK earlier in the book about how it has demonstrated the success of collaboration and cross-disciplinary work, and critical/community psychologists have done the same. This brings together people from completely different backgrounds, which cannot always be easy, but ideas around problem solving, innovation, creativity and multi-skills can be beneficial in a way that the static nature of methods and approaches mainstream psychologists use cannot be. In addition, this fits well with an intersectional approach to psychology that is becoming increasingly important in challenging structural level issues to do with oppression and equality (Rosenthal, 2016), which is at the heart of most critical/community psychology approaches.

Decolonising and deideologising psychology – Accompaniment!

One of the main epistemological considerations that is increasingly becoming a core part of what mainstream psychology or critical/community psychology can become is the importance around decolonising psychology and therefore, deideologising the status quo of psychology and other forms of psychology including community psychology. Dutta (2016, 2018) explained that decoloniality concerns repositioning colonised people and their communities as people who are the questioners, theorists, and writers of their experiences, to get a better understanding, a genuine understanding, of the histories, ontologies, and materialities of people who have been dispossessed and alienated, primarily by the powerful and dominant European-American establishment. By deideologising the status quo from hegemonic Western Eurocentric approaches in research, theory, and practice, we then go through a process that concerns challenging, unpicking, and understanding deeply held beliefs that are usually influenced by the ideologies of others around us (see Malherbe et al., 2022). This may make the interpersonal practices and subjectivities of accompaniment smoother, to better witness and advocate with the people around us (Watkins, 2015, 2021). By doing so, it highlights and interrogates the hegemonies of power ideas and power that justifies oppression, but by understanding it, may help to change it too (see Angelique, 2011).

Sonn et al. (2022b) discussed the role of knowledge production in colonising processes and the need to reclaim and reimage ways of being and doing with all parts of the world. Indeed, much has been written about these issues and some are describing the process of decolonising as a paradigm shift (Mignolo & Walsh, 2018), which may go some way to destabilising and reducing colonial systems and absence of voice from some of the most marginalised groups in society, with a view to centring the concerns and voices of people who are colonised and have been affected by colonisation. With values such as solidarity, empowerment, and voice at the heart of a critical/community psychology philosophy, collaborating with different people from different systems, nations, and societies has been vital and needs to be the life blood of a progressive and 21st century community psychology. I would posit that it needs to be a relational assemblage of accompaniments that commit to principles of reflexivity and social justice, which is central to being able to cross boundaries and disciplines to reach out and work with marginalised people (Rappaport, 1977; Montero et al., 2017; Kagan et al., 2021).

Decoloniality is being explored more than ever before within the field of critical/community psychology (see Stevens & Sonn, 2021; Kessi et al., 2021). Critical/community psychology is invoking and disrupting dominant episte-mologies that enshrine mainstream psychology and general Western thought, with a view to reframing medicalised and psychologised accounts of the most marginalised, encapsulating the political edge that is central to understanding people and to understand the psychology of people. Authors who write about decoloniality and psychology/community psychology seek to transform and centralise forgotten voices and to re-understand the entrenched Western interpretations of people's experiences, norms, and values to a position where people can speak freely about who they are, how they feel, in their contexts.

Problems and barriers for critical/community psychologists

Whilst I have briefly discussed some key tenets of critical/community psy-chologists (and there are more), earlier in the chapter, I suggested that I would focus not on regurgitating the whole history of community psychology, in all its varieties, but I would focus more on how I have seen it and what has been important to me and my interests in my work as a critical community psychologist in the UK. For example, I have not provided insights into other key areas linked strongly with community psychology such as liberation psy-chology and peace psychology as well as concepts relating to what com-munity means in all its complexities and its theories, or specific strategies, like 'communities of practice' (Wenger, 1998) or 'community development' work or listed skills and roles that critical/community psychologist might play. Also, there has not been a thorough analysis of power, politics, and eco-nomic systems that is important for many critical/community psychologists and how far one can ameliorate or transform people lives and communities for the better. There is much to write about that exists about critical/com-munity psychology and much to write about critical/community psychology to come, to fill many gaps, such as connections between critical/commu-nity psychology to sexualities, gender differences, digital technology, and interventions amongst other areas that you would expect a critical/commu-nity psychologist to be interested in. However, the queerying edge to this book would not be balanced without a review of some of the problems that have manifested within community psychology since it started arguably in the mid-1960s in the USA. Dutta (2018) points out that the foundations to the community psychology that emerged from Swampscott emerged from clinical psychology, and this is the same in the UK (Burton et al., 2007) as I have previously referred to, and other places, therefore, the very roots of mainstream community psychology stems from mainstream psychology, a psychology that is predominately white, middle-class, dominated by men, heterosexual, over the age of 40 years, the educated and wealthy (I again acknowledge that this makes up aspects of my own present identity). These characteristics continue to be what makes up the great majority of professionals, practitioners, and advocates of mainstream and community psychology, especially in the West. Can critical/community psychology really hope to decolonise and deideologise psychology without the voices of other sexualities, genders, classes, and age groups? In effect, community psychology has the same DNA as mainstream psychology and so for all its boasting of values and principles that seeks equalities and empowerment, critical/community psychology's own identities are stuck in the past and in line with mainstream psychology. Fryer and Laing (2008) have suggested that the US version of community psychology is not much different in ideology compared to the mainstream psychology that we know because it is individualistic, acritical, and not as progressive as it believes, and I have witnessed this in the UK and in other places.

One of the issues critical/community psychologist faces is the extent to which they are a collective that seeks to take action and promote social justice, wellbeing, and change for the better. If you review research papers from the mainstream community psychology journals, the methods that are generally applied in 'community work' are standard qualitative and quantitative approaches from interviews to questionnaires to surveys to regression to t-tests. Reviewing the same multitudes of papers will also reveal that whilst many seek to work with community groups, there is still predominately an element of being top-down rather than bottom-up in terms of decision-making, promoting voices, and building lasting alliances and networks. Therefore, the very essence of what you would expect any kind of critical/community psychologist to be doing in collaboration with community members is not really happening, suggesting that the 'critical' and liberatory nature of community psychology principles remain politically conservative and acritical (Fryer & Fox, 2015). This links in with an easy criticism and hypocrisy of critical/community psychology in its relationship with 'community' and what 'community' means. In my experiences of working in the community, many people in charities, organisations, councils, and government officials are eager for empowering people, making things inclusive, being artistic, and promoting voices. Yet, my experiences of working within these organisations has a paid employee, volunteer, or researcher would suggest that whilst the neoliberal and capitalist agendas are in place, then it is impossible to be in a position where you can facilitate real change, transformative change, making critical/community psychology approaches, and practices ameliorative at best, raising questions about what 'community' really means and what it means to psychologists and wider society (see Coimbra et al., 2012). I regularly saw popular and engaged community projects with marginalised groups closed down, just because funders wanted something new. If a project appeared to be too controversial, it would be dismissed. If people were eager for promotion and career progression, the focus would be on their outcomes and agenda, not the people that the project was meant to focus on (I have played a part in that with my own drive to develop as a researcher, academic and careerist). All-round, 'doing critical/community psychology' against a backdrop of neoliberal entrenchment, individualisms and ticking outcome boxes for funders was very difficult. Why would capitalist and neoliberal systems that run communities want to change things that puts them at a perceived disadvantage? This would suggest that unless critical/community psychology becomes a respected and mutually important part of psychology like the mainstream psychologies that are well established and well-funded, then critical/community psychology approaches may always run into a brick wall and cause very little change – implying that it is not just mainstream psychology that needs to change.

From an academic perspective, Parker (2007) has criticised community psychology for psychologising 'community psychology' by bringing both words together, which leads community psychologists to conceptualising the study of psychology and communities and by doing so, in effect, psychologising the individuals within it, not a lot different to mainstream psychology. Parker (2007) goes on to say that community psychology is a conservative response to the political issues within and around psychology, reducing hopes for those outside psychology and betraying those who have fought for a political agenda in psychology. I can see this in both mainstream and critical community psychology agendas, but following on from my earlier points about expectations and agendas in the community by powerful funders and leaders, they too use words like 'empowerment', 'inclusion', and 'participation' as a form of psychologising because if you do not have people attached to those words that are 'needy', 'poor', 'destitute', 'offenders', then you will not get funds. This reminds me of the dilemmas parents with autistic children face when they want their children to be formally diagnosed, they know the consequences of the label, but without the label, no help and support is provided, and when it is, the help/support/care is not the best quality. Either way, the process ignores the consequences of permanent and fixed pathologised labels that more often or not lead to people being less likely to be employed, have stable relationships, and be included in wider community groups amongst other factors. All-round, critical/community psychology has potentially enhanced the marginalisation that people face because for critical/community psychology projects to emerge and be applied, it is reliant on money, careerists, ambition, luck, and a bit of hope that people in power and the marginalised group or individuals will want to get on board in the first place.

> ## Psychology in the community rather than a community psychology
>
> Wonder
>   I am wondering about whether community psychology is just mainstream psychology in the community.
> Wander
>   I am wandering around the office where the charity I work for is based and I know the core values of community are not in play like inclusion, empowerment, and bottom-up approaches. Their idea is to take the 'day centre' concept of activities and engagement and to take it and the activities to a different location in the 'community'.
> It makes me wander back into the critical/community psychology literature where you see words like radical, liberation, peace, and solidarity, but the reality is that for those words to be real and alive for critical/community psychologists and the marginalised groups of our communities, then the psychologising of community needs to end first.

Future of community psychology

This chapter has presented my 'version' of what critical/community psychology has meant to me and some of its influences, much of which has been referred to it is fair to say has connections with different perspectives in mainstream or critical community psychology. For me, critical/community psychology provides a platform of hope that the shortcomings and old-fashioned ways of mainstream psychology can be challenged, but mainstream and critical community psychology also need to be challenged and maybe their challenge is greater. After all, the well-intentioned core values, principles, and approaches of any form of critical/community psychology are up against conservative and entrenched psychology powerbases across the world. This fits in with the neoliberal and capitalist governments agendas across many countries that only have passing reference to social justice, equality, and diversity values in their economic and political narratives, and instead prioritise medical and individualised approaches that collaborate with multi-billion-pound industries, and this will exasperate further post-Covid-19. This makes it very difficult for qualitative, creative, and dynamic approaches and setups to be founded in collaboration with marginalised people because it is not the priority of the most powerful and the elite, but then again, it never has been any different, so it should not be a surprise. The skills-based ideals from the current Conservative government in the UK, for instance, prioritises skills that are scientific, medical, and individualist in nature, ensuring that the skills, practices, and methods that might be useful for an inclusive and equal society are ignored, and that is counterproductive and counter-intuitive for a society to have a successful neoliberal culture. This can also be seen in the recent context where 'left-wing' politics has been rejected by voters, like Corbyn left-wing politics in the UK in recent years. The values of 'left-wing' politics and politicians might resonate with the values and principles of critical/community psychology, but people are not wanting it as much as one might expect. Covid-19 highlighted the inequalities of marginalised people, and therefore, provided an opportunity for the need for more critical and community based psychological approaches, this was also accompanied with the need for a vaccine to take people away from their 'imprisonment' at home. In other words, science was number one and above all things – why would helping marginalised people be more important than one's own personal and family survival? This is a harsh reflection to comprehend, but that was the mentality, it felt like the survival of the fittest, and indeed, it was marginalised people that were more likely to die from Covid-19, like with other pandemics, global crises, climate changes, wars, and economical and political fall outs.

It has been noted for some time that psychology departments, organisations, and practices are now less likely to promote alternative visions of what psychology can be especially if they seem radical and disrupt the conformity to neoliberal processes of reputation and funds. More than ever, there are less degrees, modules, practitioners, and speakers of critical/community psychology and psychology's alternatives. They have become at best a special interest topic, an opportunity for psychologists to get angry now and again, rather than making any headway in terms of penetrating, influencing, and denting the power of mainstream psychology. Additionally, whether it be mainstream or critical community psychologists, the same names dominate the space, ensuring that a patriarchal and white critical/community psychology is ever-present. Whilst more speakers and ideas are emerging in critical/community psychology from different backgrounds and communities, it is slow paced and not making headway in challenging and changing mainstream psychology. A future critical/community psychology needs to turn itself upside down and reconfigure itself into an identity that makes a real epistemological break from mainstream psychology, but in a way that is prepared to work with all kinds of psychologists, who can all bring skills, strengths, and knowledges that have the potential to genuinely change the lives of people for the better, in collaboration with them. The psychology establishment in the West will not allow a psychology like this to emerge as we know it, and it never has, it tolerates critical/community psychologists as and when convenient. This would suggest that mainstream psychology as we know it is not fit for purpose, but neither is critical/community psychology.

The contested nature of critical/community psychology, whether that be its definitions, approaches, where in the world it is, its purposes or the ever-evolving nature of community psychology (see Fryer & Laing, 2008; Dzidic et al., 2013), would imply that it will continue to be misplaced, misunderstood, meaningful, and meaningless to most people within and outside of psychology. Maybe critical/community psychologists will continue to easily criticise mainstream psychology and its individualism rather than providing a sense of what it can become by understanding people from marginalised groups from their viewpoint of their communities and world. When I consider the hardly touched definitions of mainstream psychology, untouched for over 100 years (see Chapter 2), suggesting that mainstream psychology has powered on without any real change, on the other hand, critical/community psychology has the opposite issue in that there are many definitions, which presents as something diverse, meaningful, and relational across the globe and its different contexts, but also leaves critical/community psychology with the problem that sometimes people do not know what it is and therefore is an identity crisis and is not taken seriously. Despite the hopes of critical/community psychology and its potential, it is flawed whether that be because it does not get the backing from within professional psychology, whether it be the neoliberal society we live in, or the politics of the day have not helped. But maybe the mistakes go back to when psychology started to be challenged when humanistic psychology emerged. Much of what underpins any form of critical/community psychology is what we think we understand to be 'human', so how we define who we are or who we are not in all its idio-syncrasies and diversities. To challenge psychology's power and to accentuate a psychology that can change the world for the better, a reflection is needed about what was being challenged and what are we challenging now. Critical/community psychology can be a part of that conversation and should con-sider challenging the old-fashioned definitive nature of humanistic psychol-ogy that embellishes 'human', whilst at the same time work with mainstream psychology if real change is to occur, but this is a big challenge.

In the broader scheme of things, critical/community psychology has failed in its mission. People are still not being seen in context, marginalised people are not leading research or change, people feel less empowered than ever before, protests are not working or making change happen – there is no accompaniment taking place. I do not say that critical/community psychol-ogy is a failure easily, especially when I am making a career out of it, but what does always come back to me when reflecting on this complicated area of psychology is that we must continue to have hope rather than give up, because if we know the failures, we can begin to change. A critical posthu-manities turn might help with this because the perspectives that underpin critical posthumanities might suggest that psychology needs to be relational, interconnected with people and all things at all levels, building networks and using what it available through technology to enhance our purposes within our contexts. The 'psychologists for social change' in the UK might already provide insights into what that might look like, with it being a network that is interconnected with local groups alongside psychologists that equally have social and political action at the heart of its movement (see Walker et al., 2022:34). Here, the idea is that the meaning of 'psychologists' is broad and instead it is a coalition of people from all walks of life and that is 'embodies a model of horizontal, technologically mediated, decentralised activism'. With this and the advice they provide about how to mobilise people and psychologists relating to connecting, acting, acknowledging the political, sharing skills, being brave and reflective and visionary, it is reflecting similar ideas that connect it with a critical posthumanities perspective. This gives me some hope on how critical/community psychology and mainstream psychology can go to another level in reflecting on what psychology means and what it can do, and what it can become.

Why bother with community psychology?

Wonder

I wonder about why the people I meet in the shop think I 'psychoanalyse' people when I tell them I am a critical community psychologist.

Wander

I wander through an area of Manchester, in the UK, in an area surrounded by rows of terrace housing, no front gardens, just long rows of bricks with different doors. Some doors are new, and some are damaged through past attempts to burgle the house or boarded up with aluminium sheets because they had previously been knocked down by the police to capture drug dealers. There is silence on these rows of bricks, and some rows still have cobbled roads from Victorian times, with others more modernised to tarmac. There is an eeriness about the silence, until I hear a parent shouting at a baby to shut up, and with another parent I hear a clap of a hand hitting a bum nearby. The newsagent on the end of one row is boarded up, but still open for sale, with some people marching out drunk or walking very slow with psychotic eyes. I see that some homes have very expensive cars, so maybe the owner is paid well, but likes to live in a poor area, or maybe it is stolen or loaned using money they cannot pay back. As I wander through, it feels like I am wandering again through my own streets as a little person, walking with hope that one day, I can get out of this place and not return. It makes me think about William Blake's words of 'and mark in every face I meet, marks of weakness, marks of woe' from his poem 'London', a melancholy of misery that millions of people face on a day-to-day basis. Can't psychology do anything about this?

Yes, psychology and all kinds of psychologists can do something about it, if they really want to.

Summary

In summary, this chapter has presented my version of what I understand critical/ community psychology to be and what psychology all-round means to me. It would have been easy to recount all the history, definitions, and contests between different critical/community psychologists, but other authors have done that for you, and for me. This is a reflection on an area of psychology that I have been passionate about for years, that gives me hope that psychology can be a genuine force for good, but I can only give my view on it in this book. I reflected on what critical/community psychology means to me and some 'official' versions of critical/community psychology and recognised the differences between critical/community psychology and mainstream psychology. I also considered some of the key areas of critical/community psychology and how they differentiate from the mainstream psychology that is in place. However, I also pointed out some of the big issues critical/community psychology faces in terms of applying itself with approaches that are less familiar within mainstream psychology, and acknowledged that in many respects, critical/community psychology has failed to do what it wants to do, whether through barriers out of its control or barriers that have been built up from within. For me, I still want critical community psychology, and indeed psychology in general, to change the world for the better, but it needs to go beyond simply being angry with the world and it must go beyond the discipline of psychology and draw in other voices from different disciplines and communities. Maybe psychologists need to work in a way that is never been imaginable before and we should be prepared to open our minds to this. All-round for the power that mainstream psychology is and for all the social justice principles that mainstream/critical community psychology stands for, our visibility for marginalised people is mostly non-existent and you can see that in times of crisis like Covid-19 and in day-to-day politics, policy units, hierarchies in businesses and in government and other powerful institutions. The binary between mainstream psychology and critical/community psychologies does not work and is counterproductive, but we can change this if we want to. Despite the negative ending to this chapter, I am hopeful, and we should be hopeful that we can play a part in making a difference, if we are prepared to be realistic, develop new ideas, and promote new voices from all walks of life, including and most importantly, people outside of psychology and in communities.

4 Community psychology in action – Mainstream or critical/community psychology?

In Chapter 3, I presented a narrative that was positive and negative in tone about what critical/community psychology has arguably become or what it never became in the first place. I also suggested that the future of critical/ community psychology is problematic because I cannot see how mainstream psychology is going to change. If anything, mainstream psychology will continue to become more powerful and dominate the study and practice of psychology, and critical/community psychology will continue to regurgitate its anger towards mainstream psychology and promote lots of hope about what psychology should be, without making any in-roads. But the one thing I always try and keep in mind, despite my critical tone, is 'hope'. How can we not continue to hope that mainstream psychology and critical/community psychology and other critical versions of psychology cannot become something that can change the world for the better? We must have hope, otherwise the rest of it becomes pointless.

As discussed in Chapter 3, community psychology, whether it be mainstream or critical, is a way of thinking about psychology that is different to what is familiar with mainstream psychology. This implies that critical/ community psychology is diverse and complex, rooted by the liberation and humanistic movements of the 1950s and 1960s, but overlaps in many ways with mainstream psychology too. Community psychology, in whatever form, is a critical, and to some degree, radical way of understanding, practising, and conceptualising psychology, albeit for some, it was acritical and individualistic from the start. In this respect, could critical/community psychology therefore already live up to the ideas of a critical posthumanities viewpoint, or is community psychology really just a bunch of angry psychologists who are just defining psychology in a slightly different way? After all, the people who dominate Western mainstream psychology are the same people who dominate and have dominated the development of critical/community psychology – white, mostly male, middle-class, wealthy, educated professionals, positions, and identities that are opposite to identities of many marginalised people.

To have a deeper think about critical/community psychology and its identity in more detail and following on from some of the critical reflections on

DOI: 10.4324/9781003057673-4

the future of community psychology in Chapter 3, this chapter will queery some of my own experiences and reflections of 'practising' critical/community psychology and my experiences, identity, and thoughts within those experiences. Alongside this, a critical analysis will be provided whilst drawing on other critical/community psychology studies or projects, to explore why critical/community psychology works or can work, but why also it fails to live up to its identities and values. As in earlier chapters, I recognise that my interpretations are just that, mine, and just focus on snippets of my experiences of being a critical community psychologist, and that they can be reinterpreted and contextualised in different ways, including by the people who I refer to in the vignettes and reflections. However, my main aim here is to set the scene for Chapter 5, which will present some reflections on a renewed sense of purpose for critical/community psychology and community psychologists through the lens of a 'posthuman community psychology'. But, how much do marginalised people need psychologists?

I hate psychologists

I will never forget working with one young person from a run-down and impoverished housing estate in Manchester, UK. One of my roles at the time was to help support young people who had just acquired supported accommodation, often for young people who could not live at home because of abuse, enduring mental health issues or had been involved with crime. She had just started university and she saw it as something she had to do and something that would add value to her life. She was fully aware that this would be a big challenge, not because of the usual demands of study and getting to know people in a hall of residence, but she was aware of her own mental health and wellbeing. Whilst she came across as positive, engaged, and very knowledgeable, and you could tell that this was someone who could be brilliant at whatever she wanted to be, she simply did not want to live and was always looking for opportunities to kill herself.

She always referred to this in a matter-of-fact way, often with a smile on her face, and I was never sure if this was an acceptance on her part that made her feel good or whether the smile was an awkward smile waiting for a negative or sympathetic response from me. What really struck me though was that she was very clear about what and who helped her in coping with her mental health and what did not help her.

In the years before that, I was an avid reader of Szasz and Foucault, with Szasz's provocative perspective on the social construction of mental illness being very powerful and this affected me deeply. It was no surprise to myself that regardless of changes in psychiatry over the decades, the premises that make up psychiatry, that being the values that underpin medical models, I still feel manifest themselves within medical models of care and mental health today, so I had strong views on what I think psychiatry and psychology should be (I recognise my arrogance and ignorance 15 years on).

I asked her one day, about what she thought about psychiatrists, believing that I already knew the answer, and she said they were ok and that they helped her. I said something along the lines of 'psychologists must be better' because they are less likely to be influenced by medical models of mental health for diagnosis and treatment. However, the familiar smile I was accustomed to drained away, and she looked me right in the eyes and made it very clear that she hated psychologists and that they were the worst professionals that she had worked with within the mental health systems she had engaged with.

The vignette provides me with a strong reminder that even though I was working in the community and believing that I was behaving like a 'critical/community psychologist', influenced by all those principles and values that I discussed in Chapter 3, although not deliberate, it reminds me of how arrogant psychology and psychologists can be (including my own arrogance). Here, I was thinking that I understood this person in their own complicated contexts and all I was interested in was that I was better than a mainstream psychologist and better than psychiatrists because I thought my critical way of thinking and thinking of people in context was better, meaning that I was pompous and narrow-minded. Whilst that was years ago, and I like to think I have reflected on this and become a more open-mined psychologist as a result and hopefully less arrogant, it seems to me that even when 'doing' critical/community psychology (with the vignette I was helping and supporting someone with mental health issues settle into supported accommodation), I was really being a judge in a way that was not helpful or supportive. Just because I had an anti-psychiatry stance, why should others? Who am I to say that us psychologists are better? In other similar experiences in the community, I was to find that this vignette was not a one-off. I began to generally find (and hopefully I was not looking for it) that when someone had been in contact or worked with a psychologist, those people hated them, and had better things to say about psychiatrists and other medical professionals. Even in recent years, I worked in a project in Chester (a city in the UK), with a group of adults with enduring mental health issues who faced the hard realities of poverty, and some members of the group refused to work with me because I am a 'psychologist' and it made no difference to them that I was a 'critical/community psychologist' even when I tried to explain the differences between mainstream psychology and critical/community psychology.

All round, when I was working in communities or when I talk about that work in academics settings, I point out that this was not 'happy clappy' groups of people who come together to sing hymns in the community or to attend a church tombola, common stereotypical images of community work that have been directed at me by some mainstream psychologists (and these so called 'happy clappy' activities bring happiness and communities together in many ways when they happen, and long may they continue if that is the case). However, for community workers and community members, the reality is for many that community work is gritty, smelly, dirty, aggressive, upsetting, and now and again, you might get a 'happy clappy' occasion of fun, laughter, and togetherness. Readers should not be surprised with this because what do people think the most marginalised people in society face on a day-to-day basis? Why would they have time for a psychologist who will tell them what is wrong with them and tell them what they need to do to be 'better' (but that can be helpful for some). The vignette was a young person who hated life and did not want to live in it, for reasons that were never obvious, but it was not for a psychologist of any kind to intrude on how they made sense of the world, and maybe a role of understanding, stepping back and giving 'psychology away' (Miller, 1969) would have been a better way forward.

Beyond the individual or not? What is the place of 'Other' in community psychology work?

Can you help me?

I spent some time acting as an advisor for young people aged 13–25 years in a local area of Manchester in the UK. This role was varied and involved helping young people who were homeless to get supported accommodation, helped people with issues relating to mental health, sexual health, and education, alongside setting up support and creative groups alongside health drop-in's all with a view to helping young people who had come from complex and often abusive backgrounds.

On one occasion, a male aged about 24 years contacted me to talk about whether I could help him. He had been a victim of a sex offender when he was younger, and he had found out that the person who behaved inappropriately towards him was due to be released from prison. This had a negative effect on him because whilst he felt he was bigger and stronger, the offender still had an emotional hold on him, and the news of his release took him back to those traumatic times of the abuse taking place.

He said he had contacted the National Health Service (UK) and they told him that he had to wait for over a year before any possibilities of therapy. He sought help from other places too, but he did not feel like anyone wanted to help or support him or just sit down and listen to him. He felt that his last resort was to come to this organisation which aimed to help young people.

My instinct was to help him and to reflect on what I could do to help with him about what help, or support could be possible, yet the reality was that with such a challenging and difficult situation, I did not know what to do for the best. He really wanted to talk with me and wanted me to find ways to help him.

We organised a few meetings and during those meetings, we talked through what he had experienced. He felt that using pictures to express his emotions was useful, but he rejected the idea of joining some of my group projects to talk with other men who had experienced traumatic difficulties in life.

When I reflect on this, I think that a counselling or clinical psychologist might be the better professionals to help support this man. Then again is a critical community psychologist better placed to work away from an office or clinic and look to work in creative ways rather than seeking medical or drug or psychological interventions on offer in the mainstream. Should the focus be on the individual and 'sorting out' the individual, or should the focus be on other things within that person's context and 'sorting' the issues out.

One of the main differences that critical/community psychologists claim as to why they are different to mainstream psychologists is that they view people in context. That is, the varied and complex ecologies that surround each person will affect them in direct and indirect ways, suggesting that it is not realistic to focus on the individual believing that you can change their lives for the better. This idea can be seen across other psychologies too, such as development psychology where Bronfenbrenner (1977) and other similar theorists are presented, with the classic concentric circles with the person in the middle being influenced by many diverse contextual factors. But what the vignette above makes me think about is the extent to which this is true for critical/community psychologists, so do we really see people in context? If I reflect on my own actions in the vignette, I felt like I was applying a 'person-centred' approach, whereby I showed that I cared, listened, tried to find solutions, and showed empathy to him concerning how the National Health Service let him down. Then again, how critical/community psychological was this? We spoke on a one-to-one, he felt he could only speak to me, I was presenting short-term and ameliorative solutions about how he could help himself, and in effect, I was inadvertently helping him to psychologise and individualise himself as the problem rather than focusing on ways that the contexts of his situation should and needed to change. In effect,

I was acting in a way that resonates with being a mainstream clinical or coun-selling psychologist, strands of psychology that I am readily critical about. Where was the critical/community psychologist in this vague application of a person-centred approach?

This does not just bring up issues relating to what the role, skills, and experiences a critical community psychologist should have, but it also raises questions about the standardised 'person-centred' approach that clinical and health and social care professionals are expected to apply in their work with marginalised and vulnerable people in society. In this respect, for me, it therefore brings into question what it means to be 'human' and what 'person-centred' means. When the term 'person-centred' is used, we may think of many things, and it will mean many things to different people. Key words such as 'helping', 'support', 'care', 'voice', 'needs', 'choice', 'empow-erment', 'inclusion', 'participation', and 'love' are likely to be associated with what we think is 'person-centredness' and community psychologi-cal. These are the kind of buzz words you would expect in most critical/ community psychology literature and connects to Rogers's ideas around 'person-centredness' that emerged as the 'third wave of 'humanistic psychol-ogy that developed in the 1950s onwards, which has influenced the roots of critical/community psychology in many ways. Rogers's vision was that person-centredness should not just be a helping process, but one that can produce effective change, presumably for the good of the person or people in that process. In the counselling process for instance, for one who might take this approach, this could mean providing a safe space for a client, a space where trust is developed and where a process of self-exploratory can occur, reflecting on their positionalities, identities, attitudes, values, and behaviours with a view to developing modes of coping with the issues they may face.

The aim of Rogerian person-centredness was/is to establish a congruence or genuine connection between the helper and the person they intend to help, to take away the guise of the professional mask, and to be accepting, caring, and empathetic. In this respect, my behaviour and approach in the vignette, I think, ticked those boxes. I was the helper who was in tune with who he was and how this might influence the helping process to be preventative of being judgemental and controlling and instead the aim was to be accepting. From the perspective of Rogers, person-centredness was about a 'way of being' and that genuineness should be at the core of the helping process, aiming to exclude any manipulation or coercion or pushiness for someone to change when they do not want to or need to (Rogers, 1980/1995). However, the criticism that Rogers and others faced as time went on is what I reflect on when thinking about my 'critical community psychology approach' to help-ing people. For example, Rogers faced criticism because his ideas were more philosophically based rather than set in empirical research (Ford & Urban, 1963:441), a kind of 'clinical philosophy' (Tudor & Worrall, 2006). Indeed, further criticism of this approach relates to its subjective nature and narcissism (Vitz, 1977), the process of therapy (van Belle, 1980), lack of understanding of the complexities of power (Masson, 1988), the universality of the approach and its arguably Eurocentric, patriarchal, and monocultural accelerators (Holdstock, 1993). These criticisms could be aimed at critical/community psychology approaches too, not just directed at my example in the vignette, but the same issues are within other types of critical/community psychology work as well. For example, my work with community groups (with young people and disabled people) was all facilitated with genuine empathy and determination to make a difference – but did I really think about the complications of power or my presentation as a man, white, educated without realising what effect this could have on people and collaborations? (Richards et al., 2018). Whilst 'person-centred approaches' have undergone many developments that take some of those issues on board (Tudor, 2016), and Rogers himself said that change in these approaches will always be needed, in line with the ever-changing, empathetic person that is meant to emerge from a person-centred approach, it still leaves questions of what is 'person-centred'. If the notion of 'human' is being questioned, then can it really be that easy to define what 'person-centred' really is and can we ever be 'person-centred' as psychologists or critical/community psychologists, especially when proposing a critical posthumanities perspective where there are calls for decentring the 'human'/'person'.

I have discussed in other places (Richards, 2016a, 2019) using examples of institutional abuse in care homes for people with disabilities in the UK that those 'carers', those 'professionals' who work in those settings will say they are trained in 'person-centred approaches'. They will say that they are empowering people, respecting diversity and being inclusive even when that is not the case in practice. For example, I have witnessed disabled people being told they are 'naughty' and people in care homes being told to 'shut up', so they are placed in a 'negative' category or a voiceless category. And, in US and UK contexts, the idea of 'person-centredness' is enshrined in legislation and policy, amongst other countries. In the UK, for example, in 2009, the first NHS Constitution in England stated the importance of health services prioritising the needs of patients, carers and families by emphasising that they must participate in decisions about care and treatment, and other similar policies have focused on the need for the importance of dignity and respect. Furthermore, the Health and Social Care Act 2012 in the UK enforced a legal duty that patients must be involved with their care, but then again, The Coronavirus Act 2020 empowered practitioners to decide what level or if any care could be given to chosen, selected people, so 'person-centredness' is an important concept for people and politicians, but how this is applied and defined is more complicated. Similarly, the Health Foundation (2018) emphasised the need to work collaboratively and help people make informed decisions and NHS England (2022) make clear that 'person-centred care' aims to support people to make choices and manage their own health and care, and that it should be tailored to the needs of the person in collaboration with healthcare professionals. This is underpinned by the 'Five Year Forward

View' (2014) policy that aims to change the relationships between the NHS and people. The vision of this emerged because it was identified that whilst there are better scientific outcomes such as better patient satisfaction and cancer and cardiac rates are better, the policy recognised that the needs of their patients are changing, technology is changing and the demands for services are building. It pledges to help patients have greater control for their care and back nation campaigns relating to obesity and alcohol and aim for more control to be given to local governments and charities (very much relating to a Conservative agenda in the UK). The policy also pledges to break barriers down for how care is provided, and it appears indecisive about a 'one size fits all' approach to care opposed to something to something individual and specific for different people. All-round, the policies are top-down, individualistic, and focused on individual change.

With 'person-centred' care and approaches being universal in health and social care discourses in the UK and other countries (Godfrey et al., 2018), alongside changes in methods, attitudes, and policies since those earlier days of Rogers and others, it seems to me that person-centredness has lost meaning. Its application is complicated and maybe does not consistently fulfil the role of empowering people as much as we like to believe especially for marginalised groups ignoring the relational and diverse nature of people. There are underpinnings of the biomedical approach to health and social care, which has traditionally been seen as a source for where patient/clients voices are not being heard, choice being taken out of their hands and the approach to mental health, for instance, mental health has primarily been treated as a physical condition. Incorporating person/patient-centred approaches into biomedical care was an attempt to steer away from cure over care (Leplege et al., 2007), with the aim to strengthen congruent relationships and empathy, working with families, loved ones and carers. Whilst in the UK and other parts of the West there is a combined biomedical-person-centred approach established, with the best intentions to help people feel better and to be less poorly, the reality is that there are major issues that come with the operationalising of health care systems that postulate that person-centred care should be at the heart of what they do, despite the issues with this approach. For example, the National Health Service in the UK, care and education institutions and individual carers and practitioners that are rhizomatic through the care system, that would claim to be 'person-centred' without fully understanding what the 'person' is because there is a lack of voice, lack of bottom-up approaches and no appetite for transformative change. Similarly, humanistic psychology has lost meaning (arguably decades ago) by being part of the mainstream psychology and with critical/community psychology approaches also attesting to being humanistic and person-centred in nature, it too has lost meaning and a sense of vision of how it can make a difference in people's lives. Mainstream and critical/community psychology have both taken aspects of the humanistic psychology ideas and sucked it up to form their own positions and ideas about how to practice and apply psychology, but without really thinking about what 'human' means. This analysis links with a critical posthumanities outlook and an outlook that might help critical/community psychology and psychology in the mainstream. For example, rather than focusing on the 'problematic' individual and their immediate context with ameliorative actions and solutions, a decentred approach of assemblages to how we understand humans might go some way in us rethinking and revisioning what psychology can become, that is both mainstream and critical/community psychology (see Deleuze & Guattari, 1987; Braidotti, 2013; Goodley & Runswick-Cole, 2016).

I have provided quite a bit of analysis based on one vignette alone, but my reflections connect with my other experiences of work in the community and my analysis of critical/community and mainstream psychology literature. If we are to say that we view the person in context, then we need to know what we mean by 'person' in all its ambiguities, rather than just go straight to the contexts or straight into analysing individualised behaviour. Critical/community and mainstream psychologists need to work on questions on what it means to be human because this relates to questions concerned with standardising care and whether you can train people to be 'person-centred' with so much difference or does the delivery of care really mean people are empowered and have really made decisions about their lives. Gibson et al. (2021) provided a critique of 'person-centred' care and explored the possibilities of 'becoming' rather than being positioned in a way that is fixed, prescribed and dictated by 'experts'. They suggest that the 'means-to-an-end' approach can only enhance the overpowering influences of biomedical models, the objectification of the body, then the binary of body-mind, expert-novice, carer-patient, will continue to deindividuate people and ignore context. Psychologists of all kinds need to be thinking about this in their research, practices and how they identify as a psychologist and citizen in the world so that psychology can emerge as something that is not just person-centred rhetoric and tokenistic.

Whose justice are community psychologists fighting for?

The 'handicapped'

I helped to co-create and co-facilitate an advocacy project that involved working with adults with intellectual disabilities (referred to earlier in the book) to develop some creative training with a view to challenging entrenched disablist attitudes. On one occasion, we negotiated with the landlady of a local public house about presenting our work to some of the local customers and invited guests. No doubt that one of the main reasons was she agreed to do it was to draw in more customers to buy beer, but it suited our purpose of working within the community with local people to challenge stereotypes around disabilities.

The local mayor was invited with some of her colleagues from the council, alongside a Member of Parliament, and the event was very well attended. The atmosphere was good and positive, and the actors were looking forward to showcasing their scenes and poetry and to express their opinions about their experiences of disablism.

The group presented their work, which included emotional accounts of falling in love with members of the same sex, and stories of crime against them and of carers not treating them the way they wanted to be treated. The stories and short drama scenes were powerful pieces, but it was quite clear that the audience were uncomfortable. People were cringing, almost hiding their faces and some were clearly keen to leave this part of the public house to go to the bar. The people who led the charity that housed the project were also uncomfortable, and this is primarily because they saw this event as an opportunity to make 'important connections' and therefore the content of the work by the group was being frowned upon. I got the impression that the audience were expecting to see performances that were 'nice' and 'hopeful' rather than creativity stories that depicted the real intersubjective experiences of disabled people's lives.

Once the group had finished their performances, the mayor made a short speech about how much she enjoyed being there, although this was not so apparent during the performances. However, during her short speech, she referred to the group by using the word 'handicapped'. In the UK context, words like 'handicapped', 'spastic', and 'retard' are considered out of date, offensive words are related specifically to people who might now be described as someone with intellectual disabilities/ learning disabilities/learning differences amongst other terms. The group of performers were outraged with the use of this word, and I challenged the mayor about this use of language. The reaction was not positive from her or the audience members from the charity, and the Member of Parliament was clearly uncomfortable about the reaction from the use of the word 'handicapped'. The audience in general did not consider why this word would be considered offensive and seemed to contradict what the group were trying to do, that is challenge disablism and promote the voices of disabled people.

My relationship with the charity I was attached to at the time was not quite the same again after, and I soon resigned. They placed importance on not 'embarrassing' the organisation over challenging people in people who were, deliberate or not, disablist. I can empathise with that situation, organisations are dependent on goodwill, council funds, and want to be seen to be in line and professional, yet, that stance also means what needs to be challenged or changed, goes unchallenged and unchanged.

In Chapter 3, I commented on how social justice is important to me and many critical/community psychologists, and it will be important for many mainstream psychologists too. Nonetheless, as we have seen with protest movements such as the Black Lives Movement and MeToo campaign (2018–2022), shouting out for change and promoting voices is significant, but does it really make a difference and force transformative change? My example in the vignette would suggest that what comes hand-in-hand with fighting for social justice is that no matter how much shouting you do, with the hope that you can make a difference and make change happen, it arguably never really makes a difference for marginalised people. The barriers they face are so powerful, which is concerning because the battles that marginalised groups and others have fought for in our lives and history, to be able to have a voice, seem at times empty and hopeless.

The social justice issue in the vignette concerns disabled people wanting to promote their voices through creative means within the local community alongside officials who ran the city of Manchester, UK. They used their time, unpaid, to prepare for the work they wanted to present, but were made to feel uncomfortable and different in a way that was negative and disempowering, in a space where they expected the opposite. The people in power and the people more concerned with image were uncomfortable and derogatory towards the group. My position must also be questioned. Was I the hero who stood up for the group or was I the one who exasperated the alienation? Whatever way you look at it, I do not think social justice prevailed because the voices of the group were ignored, we were not asked to go back, and the people in power were embarrassed about how they looked rather than being touched by the emotive, creative stories, and expertise of the group.

Reflecting on this, with social justice being a core value of what critical/community psychology is meant to be about, in comparison to mainstream psychology, it would suggest that critical/community psychology has acted to some extent as a voice or provided a space for marginalised people to have a voice, but that real social justice change has not happened. If you consider the wider literature on 'social justice' issues within mainstream or critical community psychology, it has been a talking shop for social justice issues and that is as far as it goes and not touch the surface in one of its ultimate goals towards transformative change. If I take my own work, I have worked with homeless people, disabled people, people with mental health issues, people in poverty and used a range of methods to do this, in the name of 'critical/community psychology' and its principles (Richards et al., 2018, also see Simpson & Richards, 2018). But the homeless are still homeless, the people with mental health issues are still tortured, and disabled people are still disabled. Whilst I have put together competent and creative pieces of work that have brought some happiness, some success, and ticked boxes for me within my job, the social justice issues have not been resolved. Yes, I am realistically not going to change the world or revolutionise people's lives on my own to make things better for people, then again, if critical/community psychology is all about difference and changes, then why am I not doing that alongside my allies in critical/community psychology?

The vignette explains some of the reasons relating to structures and power bases in place, which will only allow voices of marginalised people to talk and express their experiences to an extent and in certain ways that suit. If presenting a social justice issue to funders in a way that is scientifically evidence based, that does not sound too critical or radical, then their voices are heard more. Once you relay difference over the status quo, power bases are nervous because they recognise, they are part of the problems the marginalised face in the first place. Could this also be the reason why some critical/community psychologists tend to do 'psychology in the community' using traditional, scientific methods of surveys, questionnaires, and quantitative analyses, to fit in rather than be different when difference and change is what critical/community psychologists tend to look for or implement? Are we as critical/community psychologists concerned too much or sound too radical, which might lead to us not being accepted in that community setting by the power structures or even achieve ethical approval for daring to think of new ideas or new methods? The systems that critical/community psychologists work in profess that they want change and want their marginalised groups to be happier and have better lives, but those same systems expect apolitical and acritical methods, practice, and applications, which ensures that the social justice they want to resolve can never really be resolved.

On a wider scale, I noted in Chapter 3 that a further problem with thinking about social justice issues is that different cultures, countries, and groups have different expectations of what social justice is and how to resolve the issues, for example, for claiming to promote equal opportunities for all to the opposite where there are very limited equal opportunities for all such as LGBTQIA+ rights that vary across the world. To promote social justice, it must be much more than just protesting in the streets – does that ever bring change? There must be a mutual sense of injustice that cuts across policy, legislation, sharing of resources and support and expertise, but also mutual understanding that intersects across class, age, gender, sexualities, and ethnicities, to be able to recognise our multiple and complex identities whilst living in the same world. Overall, critical/community psychology and critical/community psychologists cannot be responsible for changing the world, alone, but whilst 'change' and social justice are at the core of what critical/community psychologists are meant to be about, and transformative change has not happened, then critical/community psychology is a major failure.

Creative interventions – Going beyond 'psychology in the community'

Power of creativity and voice

I remember one of the most energised workshops I facilitated in the community. This workshop aimed to facilitate some generic sexual health work I was funded to do for groups of young men aged 13–25 years in some of the poorest areas of Manchester, UK. This involved developing dialogues around contraception usage, following on from other workshops relating to 'equal opportunities', 'diversity', and 'masculinity and identity'.

The boys came in at 9 am in the morning, about 15 of them, all very rowdy, smelling of smoke, and hints of cannabis reeked from them, with some young men looking 'spaced out' as they said hello to me. They always smelt like they had not washed and always had crumbs down their clothes or bits of tobacco, so the smell of the room very quickly changed from being rather clinical with no smell to a room of distinctive boyish smells.

I let them know that we would be following on from the discussions we had in previous weeks on sexual health and related subjects, and I created a quiz for them to do on types of contraception. However, the workshop ended up being very different from normal. They kept talking to one another and did not want to do the quiz and it all felt a bit awkward for me. In the end, I just went around and collected all the quizzes in and just sat down at the front looking at them. Eventually, the noise started to quieten down and there was an awkward silence in the room from being very loud. During the 'noise', I noticed that one young man, who had been very quiet and unassuming, and who was sat down on his own, was getting some grief from some of the boys. In the end, this made me go over to him and ask if he was ok and he just nodded in a way that made me feel that he was not ok, but he was not interested in my support. I did remain worried because the boys were making fun of him too much. When the awkward silence came, I eventually said to the group that there is no point in me carrying on because they did not want to do it, so I was happy to just sit here and just talk. Some of the boys looked at each as if to say, 'this is a bit weird'. This was then followed by some banter, and they liked doing this with me because they do not expect the 'teacher' to talk at 'their level'. But then this was followed by another awkward silence and my brain was on full alert that I needed to think of something to do that appeased them in a way where I was doing the job I was meant to do.

Then something extraordinary happened and I have never forgotten it. The man who appeared to have been bullied and quiet, suddenly in this awkward silence, started to hum quietly what sounded like very fast words, which gradually got louder. My initial thoughts (stupid when I look back now) were that he was having some kind of fit because he was shaking as he started to hum and speak fast. The other young men started to smile and look at me, thinking 'what the fuck is going on here', all of us wondering what was going on. I thought the bullying from before was having a nasty effect on this boy. Then unexpectedly, he started to sing and rap, using words that I could never remember because he was rapping so fast, but I heard of a lot of phrases such as 'mother fucker', 'weed', 'booze', 'shagging', and themes about family life, school, his hatred for teachers, and not having any money. His rapping went on for about 2/3 minutes and the mood in the room went from awkwardness and witnessing something bizarre to happiness and witnessing something special. The faces of the boys changed to faces that looked like they now respected this boy. When he stopped rapping, he was out of breath and smiling because everyone was cheering him and clapping. It was such a beautiful moment. When that cathartic outpouring ended, another boy, one of the boys who had been making fun of the rapper, just suddenly started to do exactly the same for two minutes. Now the atmosphere was electric and joyous for everyone and people from rooms outside were peering in to see what was going on. Again, the rapping was fast and covered the same kind of subjects as the previous rapper. Quite simply these boys made this workshop their own about themselves and about their lives, and this is what I always wanted the workshops to be about, not about me, but all of us. When this rapper stopped, he received a round of applause and cheers. Then one of the men said, 'hey sir, it's your turn' and I said, 'fuck off' and we all burst out laughing and we all went out together for a break.

(Adapted from a blog by Richards, 2014b)

This workshop was special to me because despite the rap performances being in a language that was fast, full of swear words, sex, and violence, and some of the language was politically incorrect, the compositions the boys created were emotional, edgy, and real to them and to everyone in the room. Their creativity reflected their ambiguous contexts where they struggled to be able to celebrate and express their identities. However, in a participative, free-flowing workshop, where they made their own choices, the boys were able to express themselves and feel happy to be able to be what they wanted to be in a safe space. Some may say I was simply a bad facilitator because it looked like I lost control, but my aim was never to control and instead try to be collaborative and be adaptive, so moments of individualism within this collective space could happen. These boys already knew about contraception and sexually transmitted infections, and I was never going to 'teach' them much anyway, but what they did do was learn about life from each other in their own way and this kind of reflectivity in their contexts is rare. Doing this job was great fun because there was much to learn and much to laugh about, and for me, this was community work at its best. What was great about working in the community was not the pre-planned activities, and they are likely to change and adapt anyway, it is when you witness something unexpected, and this somehow transcends beyond what you imagine is going to happen.

Similar to other examples I have provided, despite the power of voice coming through, this group of boys were still going to go back to their lives and face the same challenges, rendering my interventions as pointless in terms of making a real difference. That being said, it did help me to reflect on this creativity and imagination and my frustrations with mainstream community psychology, that for me lacks creativity, alternative methods, and bottom-up approaches within studies and projects that take place in the name of 'community psychology'. If you review the main community psychology journals, based mostly in Europe and the USA, with editorial teams made up mostly of Europeans and Americans (but becoming more diverse), they do not present the many thousands of papers and projects in other disciplines and professions that exist that are creative, innovative, and exciting, and instead, most papers are made up of surveys, questionnaires, quantitative approaches, and methods that feel mainstream psychology. The same papers will refer to 'critical/community psychology approaches', but the studies are almost exclusively top-down, and the methods/tools/resources are 'given' to the community to use during the course of the study, and then that it is that. This means no changes, no voices, no innovations, and no creativity emerge, and this is disappointing, when you think of this in the context of the spontaneity and the beauty of what was presented in the vignette.

It would suggest that mainstream psychology is just 'psychology in the community', taking its work into the community and the tools that go with it, which seem to be a long way from the innovative and value-driven community psychology that I dreamed about what community psychology can become, with emphasis on bottom-up approaches and voices of marginalised people. To what extent are people who are in extreme poverty, homeless, sectioned in mental health institutions or abused or imprisoned, going to be interested in surveys, experiments, questionnaires, interviews, focus groups, and similar inaccessible tools? Most would not be interested it is fair to say because they do not have the means, the time, or the concern to please a well-intentioned, well-paid critical/community psychologist, who wants to spend time doing what many mainstream psychologists do – pathologise, individualise, and psychologise. Therefore, the use of appropriate, empowering tools and methods is important to help make the voices of marginalised people more accessible and more heard in the work and processes of being any kind of psychologist. This might sound obvious, but why is it not so obvious in mainstream critical/community psychological work?

Being intersectional and multidisciplinary

Sitting on Father Christmas's knee

I was invited to a Christmas party one year along with a group of people who I was supporting who had intellectual disabilities. The party was an 'official' one in the sense that a random, established motor insurance company wanted to do a good deed and provide some money with the intention that local people with intellectual disabilities would have a chance to have a party with food and a dance at Christmas.

We arrived at the local community centre and were welcomed into the space, and we went and sat down around a table in the middle of the room. What was noticeable was that the respite workers, social workers, residential workers, and carers, all pitched themselves around the circumference of the room, with all the people they cared for, the ones with intellectual disabilities, placed in the centre around about 10 large round tables with chairs. I chose not to do the same because why would I not sit with the people I came with?

The insurance people who came on the day, to see how their funds were being spent, put on some Christmas cracker hats, with a bit of tinsel around their necks and came around, poured drinks (non-alcoholic) and gave out party food. I recall that one of them started to pour out a drink for me and was nodding his head and smiling at me as he did it, without asking whether I wanted a drink or not, and not sure why he was smiling at me. I came to realise that he and his fellow workers were working their way around the room and were doing the same to the other people in the middle, so I am guessing he had labelled me with 'intellectual disabilities' because I was sitting with people with intellectual disabilities.

Two other things struck me about the event that was taking place. First, when some of the 'disabled' people started to shout and laugh loudly, there were tuts from the people around the outside of the room, and the insurance people were asking people to calm down and not 'spoil' it for others. The voices were just excited voices who were pleased to be at a party – are parties for making noises anyway? The second thing that struck me was that this party was not about making the 'disabled' feel better and grateful that they had been given this 'opportunity', but it was clearly about making the insurers feel good and the carers feel good that they could 'release' those in their care out of their care for a little while.

Soon after I had been labelled with intellectual disabilities with the insurer's eyes, once he poured the drink out for me, someone put some loud music on with Christmas songs playing, and a moment later, a man dressed as Father Christmas came into the room, clearly an older man dressed up. After some 'Ho Ho's', the people in the centre were then invited to come up to speak to Father Christmas and a number of them were invited to sit on his knee. To be clear, that is adult men, women, and other genders, mostly over the age of 50 were being asked to sit on Father Christmas's knee. Some were excited to do this, and others were clearly very uncomfortable, and they were labelled 'party poopers'. Eventually, I was asked to go up and sit on his knee, and I was nearly dragged by my arm to do it by one of the workers, and I politely moved my arm away, and unsurprisingly, I said 'no' and I became a party pooper.

I remember vividly sitting there thinking, 'what the fuck is going on here .... am I in a parallel world?'. It made me think, is this what it was like when rich people paid to visit the 'mad' people in Bedlam? ('Bedlam' was an asylum for the mentally ill in London, UK, at the 'St Mary of Bethlehem' hospital, where the wealthy would pay to visit the mentally ill for their entertainment in the 1600s and 1700s).

When I was working with this group of people, on a day-to-day basis, I felt that I was applying a critical/community psychology approach or practice that was underpinned by values, empowerment, inclusion, and promotion of marginalised voices. With this group, I would participate in creative activities, go on day trips, read poetry, and challenge disablist thinking through great debates, amongst other things. I was playing the role as support worker, psychologist, researcher, carer, friend, and other roles that epitomises the multiple and diverse roles that critical/community psychologists can play, beyond the classic image of a psychology being about white men in white coats in a laboratory of rats testing their behaviour. Yet, this vignette also highlighted the problem of not doing the norm, which is what professionals or people in those roles I have highlighted, are expected to follow. How different would the experience for me and the people I was working with if I had stood on the outside, went around pouring drinks like disabled people were not capable of doing it themselves or if I had decided to sit on an old man's knee, a stranger dressed as a pantomime type character? By becoming 'Other' alongside the people with intellectual disabilities, I could see issues to do with power and empowerment, social justice and inclusion, and dismissal of diversity and choice. The workers, carers, and insurers in the room no doubt would have felt that they were doing a good deed, and there is no doubt that they wanted to do something that was caring and special for the people in the room. However, there were limited choices, limited decisions to be made, no sharing of expertise, no control, and the identities of people were stifled into one group, ensuring that diversity and difference was controlled or dismissed, all this in one event, in one moment in time (Richards et al., 2018).

In this example, there was an absence of voices, and whilst this cannot be down to my role as a critical/community psychologist entirely, it makes me reflect on what 'Other' means in the context of critical/community psychology. If critical/community psychology concerns social justice, empowerment, inclusivity, and participation, then how easy it to do this in the complex roles and positioning of critical/community psychologists? How far can we claim that we are promoting the voices of Others and at one with Others when we contribute, inadvertently or not, to ensuring that 'Other' remains 'Other'? To understand these processes more, most critical/community psychologists would agree that working across and within disciplines and to be intersectional in their work, is an all-encompassing way to understand people in all their differences and circumstances. If a group of youth workers had been running the event in the vignette, would the outcomes and setup have been the same? If a group of professional artists had worked with the people in the group, would sitting on Father Christmas's knee be the central activity? My point is that the event was a community version of a laboratory setup or the setup you would expect in a prison or mental health hospital, in that it was controlled, the people were infantilised, objectified, and watched, in ways that other professionals might have avoided.

To recognise people in their contexts and how these contexts psychologise and individualise those people, psychology needs to come from within its psychologies and be prepared to be a multidisciplinary psychology. This means looking from within and going beyond what they know to be 'truth' and open their minds up to progressive and radical perspectives from any discipline that works for the communities they work with. Indeed, there are more bridges being built across disciplines, albeit with a view to strengthen funding opportunities and having greater kudos in the academic context's researchers want to be in. But whilst it is not done with full on altruism, recognising strengths and the skills of all professionals, clinicians, and people in the communities it might go some way in breaking down barriers to participation, if we are prepared to share power and decision making with all.

Decolonising and deideologising community psychology

Deideologising myself

I mentioned in my introduction to this book that I came from a Roman Catholic background, a childhood experience of contradictions, hypocrisies, and misuse of power. That being said, there was a period of time during my teenage years where I found solace in being a 'believer', and this led to widespread mockery from friends, school, and the local church. The more you were associated with it, the more expectations were placed on you to be a good person, and any sense of spirituality and being at peace bought more attention and more focus on whether you were being good or not and meeting norms, values, and expectations of society and what suited the powerful figures around me.

I was to learn later that whilst established religions and beliefs in gods are important to people and help people in a lot of ways, my experiences of religion caused me more problems. My introduction to Marx made me realise that these systems are built on similar systems you find in neoliberal ideologies and in psychology, patriarchal, money-focused, and they pick out what marginalised groups are worthy of their attention, as and when.

My critical views went further when I started university when I started to read and spend a lot of time thinking about the works of Foucault and Szasz, and this was taken further when I started to work within marginalised groups and within powerful systems that would pride themselves on doing everything, they did in the interests of the marginalised groups they served. But they never really made a transformative difference and, indeed, made things worse in many ways (and I have played my part in that too in obvious and less obvious ways).

I feel like I have spent the past 30 years going through periods of purging reductionist and conservative ways of thinking about people and their contexts that enshrined me from a conservative religious upbringing to a radical posthuman thinking that freed my mind and made me happier in a way than ever before. I feel that I am constantly reideologising myself, which can leave me with a confusing, contradictory, and hypocritical set of morals and values that I practice and not other times, but I feel that this also helps me to be the best psychologist I can be, so I am constantly in flux, becoming a new psychologist all the time – at least I hope so (see Drake et al., 2022 for a discussion for a radical decolonialisation of psychology).

My queerying reflections on my own changing ideologies and identities, whether they have been forced upon me or whether I have acquired them as I develop and grow or hit dead ends or make mistakes, has helped me to think about psychology's ideologies. In Chapter 2, I presented a positivist-laden history of modern psychology and how it still permeates through to the present contemporary psychology as the 21st century progresses, but I have also written about how critical/community psychology has not been much different in certain respects. One of the key similarities about mainstream psychology and critical/community psychology is the colonial and white-dominated feel to all parts of psychology (acknowledging again that as the narrator of this book I too link in with this and may write with that gaze, intentional or not).

The reflections above have led me to go back time and time again to the work of Fanon (1952/1967), particularly when thinking about the powerful grip of colonialism on psychology. The insights he brought relate to the need for a decolonial turn in psychology, and this has been very slow in the context of psychology all-round, but for any form of psychology to be able to claim that it is then about empowering people and shared expertise and genuine participation, that Fanon proposed, but is still not in place, that is the need for psychology to be a decolonial and transdisciplinary practice that links with activism and praxis and other similar disciplines such as sociology, political theory, and philosophy (Maldonando-Torres, 2017). In this respect, decolonising psychology in all its forms is vital because of the privileged position that white, Westernised perspectives continue to hold. A privileged position that produces knowledge (Sonn, 2016) that cannot be in tune with the values set out by most critical/community psychological approaches because how can we ever know and understand poverty, poor health and abuse and other serious issues, for instance, that people face, with the narrow gaze of whiteness and privilege.

We already know that mainstream psychology has drawn on theories such as Social Darwinism and eugenics and this has historically been used to categorise and marginalise people. This has linked negatively on races and aspects of this can also be connected back to intelligence which I discussed earlier in the book, ensuring that mainstream psychology like other institutions in society as a poor history in understanding race and issues to do with colonialisation like many established institutions in our societies. Historically, psychology has defended concepts such as 'survival of the fittest' and still uses the mind and brain as a way to differentiate people, with marginalised people continuing to be on the negative side of this, so a decolonial turn would help move away from psychology's obsession with the individual level of analysis and draw on the wider economic and political contexts. To do this, psychology needs to be turned upside down and reconsidered because the oppressed need to emerge as equal agents of change that is a collective of people that is driven by activism and political organising (see Dutta, 2016, 2018). Whilst liberation, postcolonial, and feminist forms of politicised psychology have been around for decades, bringing a critical and social focus to psychology and explore the power relations from within psychology, there is still much more to be done. A decolonial turn that is intersecting and diverse and contextualised has the power to activate psychologists into turning to more creative and innovative ways to promote voices and conscious raising to lead to social action.

My vignette alludes to aspects of my deideologisation and a vague route to my own conscious raising to broaden my mind to help my ideas and view of the world intersect and take action. That process of change is something that resonates with the process that is needed to decolonise psychology and previously, I have made comparisons with mainstream and critical community psychology not being a lot different to mainstream psychology, and so they too need decolonise if real social action can be done. To do this, and Fanon and others have written about this, is that knowledge exchange and production needs to take place with people's lived experiences, intersubjective and intricate or broad and big, it all counts and there is a need to be reflective on our uses of power, resources, judgements, and labelling and why we do this. This conscious raising (also see Freire, 1970) brings realities for marginalised people to the forefront and for a socially just society to emerge and for a socially just psychology to emerge, we must know the lives of the most marginalised if we have a genuine view to make collective change.

Powerbases in critical/community psychology – Disguised mainstream psychology?

Pre-2014 – Medical doctor experiences

I will never forget an experience I had with a dentist when I was in college, aged about 20 years old. It was a private dentist that I had attended a few years before, when I was in agony and had to have a tooth taken out. I felt obliged to stay and go regularly, especially as I did not have to pay the huge sums many have to pay because there was an exemption because I was studying.

One day, I attended an appointment, and a new set of dentists had taken over the business. I was wearing a baseball hat and sports clothes, so felt quite relaxed and comfortable before having a dentist stick their instruments into my mouth. It is worth noting that in the UK, the image of a young man wearing baseball hat and sports clothes is often stereotyped as being troublesome, criminal, and even dangerous.

I walked into the clinical room and was told to take my hat off and he commented along the lines of 'are you scared stolen goods will fall from your hat' (because he thought I was wearing the hat to hide stolen goods). Whilst he might have been joking, from his own perspective, there was an air of judgement and labelling by this dentist, which is still something I think about today, that felt real, even that it was not real. It was only when I said to him that I was currently studying my A-levels that his tone became a bit more respectful.

Post-2014 – Medical doctor experiences

There were several occasions, similar in nature, over the following years that felt the same when speaking to health care professionals, but this was to change some 10–15 years after.

Since achieving a PhD, the attitude, tone, and behaviour of health care professionals have changed for me when I have needed their services. For example, it is now common for a GP to sit up straight when they read my notes and see that I am a doctor. They are more relaxed, friendly, and talk to me like we are old friends. A sharp contrast to the attitudes I experienced as a young man. Although now I attend a different dental practice these days, but I will still dress in a relaxed fashion, and even that my personal details state 'doctor', I have the impression that the dentist thinks I am making it up, no doubt because I am not wearing tweed, or a cravat, or sound posh, I therefore cannot possibly be a doctor.

In my introduction to this book, I introduced that I would be 'queerying' myself and that there would be a critical autoethnographical twist to the narrative, to acknowledge that before I judge others, I need to look at myself and reflect on my positions and identities that not just influence the narrative but also my practices and behaviours when working with people. There will be aspects of my personal reflections about my positions, identities, and approaches within the stories I have presented that some will say is a heroic discourse or a fake humbleness in what I do. Nevertheless, I acknowledge things as they happen and as I reflect on them and I know that my status as a man, white, educated, and being a 'doctor' gives me opportunities and a 'foot in the door' in different aspects of life, and this can be seen in the example above where the whole experience of my relationship with medical professionals completely changed purely based on my title as 'doctor'. I have also previously mentioned that this 'power' has led to people not wanting to work with me in the community because of their fears and anger towards psychology and psychologists.

The vignette is a more recent reminder to me about the power of psychology, and psychologists, and related professions and disciplines and what this means when working with marginalised groups and institutions. I have consistently been critical of mainstream psychology, mostly because of its powerful position, yet are critical/community psychologists really any different when it comes to power? Whilst we have the word 'psychology' and 'psychologist' attached to us, it does not matter what values or what position you hold within the discipline, you are still likely to have 'power' over people, whether it be in day-to-day life or over 'younger' psychologists or over marginalised people. Does that mean, inadvertently or not, that as critical/community psychologists, as we are preaching that we are value-driven, bottom-up psychologists, determined to make psychology an equal and diverse space, do we realise we are carrying the fleas of what we are challenging and spreading the power, inequalities, and exclusionary practices that encompass many aspects of psychology on marginalise groups?

The vignette below reminds me that mainstream psychology is very powerful and dominant, but it will remain so if not challenged and unpicked, and seeks to equally work with other psychologies that might challenge mainstream psychology:

'Community psychology' does not exist?

In recent years, I prepared a small research project which involved working with different genders, mostly over the age of 50 years, in a poor area of Liverpool, UK. The project involved some drawing and a focus group that explored the relationship between disabilities and health. All in all, it was a relatively straightforward piece of work that I had done in other places and the participants were looking forward to expressing themselves through their voice and through drawings. To be able to start this project and collect data, I needed ethical approval to make sure the study was competent and safe to do, like it is necessary for all kinds of research. The ethics committee that was to judge my ethics application were mostly made up of mainstream psychologists and other empirically driven academics.

I eventually was sent my feedback, and the feedback in parts was fair and you persevere in getting the amendments done so that you can achieve ethical approval and start the project. However, one of the last comments that was made on the feedback was 'delete references to community psychology because it does not exist'. Naturally, as someone who has been a flag bearer for critical/community psychology for a long time, I was not happy with this comment. I contacted the Chair and made it clear about why critical/community psychology does exist, and I did receive an apology and the proposed amendment in deleting reference to community psychology was rejected.

Why would mainstream psychologists say critical/community psychology does not exist? By then, community psychology was an established Section of the British Psychological Society in the UK, and decades of publications, projects, and activities had long taken place in the UK and around the world. Whatever the answer might be or what the motivations the person/people who had made that comment, it was a stark reminder to me that if we have discord within critical/community psychology itself, mainstream vs. critical, then that is not even half the problem when it comes to facing up to a mainstream psychology that does not want or feel it needs critical/community psychology.

Summary

This chapter provided some reflections on community psychology in action and highlighted the complexities of 'doing' community psychology, at least from my experience. Whilst the reflections and insights are just about me and my experiences and might present as a form of self-flagellation or a 'mea culpa' (an acknowledgement of one's own fault, a term used in the Roman Catholic Latin mass), all of them relate to issues that are relevant to critical/community psychologists. They highlight that if you have a discipline that is defined in many ways, with many roles, many issues to do with power and building alliances, then doing critical/community psychology is very hard, and possibly counterproductive, in a way that mainstream psychology is counterproductive with similar issues.

My final vignette was a final reflection in this chapter on what I and other critical/community psychologists face and that is this continued binary of mainstream psychology vs. other psychologies that challenge mainstream psychology. The reality is that neither side of the binary works for marginalised people, ensuring that if psychology in all its entities continues in this way, then psychology as it stands cannot continue as we know it because people in our communities will not recognise psychology as a force for good and change, which most marginalised groups want and need. If this is the case, then new ideas, perspectives, and imagination need to be explored. This chapter has focused on my practices, behaviours, and reflections on doing 'critical/community psychology' and not so much a reflection on how critical posthumanities fit into this. However, with those reflections in mind, the next chapter will present a set of ideas of how mainstream psychology and critical/community psychology can emerge as something that might help to overcome some of these issues by putting forward some reflections on what a 'posthuman community psychology' could bring.

5 Posthuman community psychology

Wonder

I am wondering what it would be like if mainstream, community, and critical psychologies did not exist anymore.

Wander

I wander back to a recent memory of when I went down to Strawberry Fields in Liverpool, UK, with my son in March 2022, located around the corner from where John Lennon, the 'working class hero' lived in his youth, and we played in the park nearby. And I wander back to that week, the same week my dad passed away unexpectedly, and the world changed forever. He hated conflict and fighting and was always kind, not expecting anything in return. It made me wander through my brain, like a time traveller, and think about many things, including my journey as a psychologist. Why did I come to hate so much of what mainstream psychology represented and why have I become a critic of psychology, but still maintain hope and belief that psychology can be a social movement for good? Why are critical and community psychologists so angry, hateful, and can never provide any real sense of change, action, and hope that psychology and the world can change?

I think of me, where I have come from, where I am now and where I could be one day, the good, the bad, and the in-between. My dad changed my world, and if one man can change my world and I have changed the world for others, imagine what it would be like if everyone could be kind and had common purposes – imagine what psychology could become and how it could really change the world.

DOI: 10.4324/9781003057673-5

Every time I hear the song 'Strawberry Fields Forever' by the Beatles, I get this image of a field of red, with lots of strawberries to pick and eat, on a nice summer's day, and I can almost smell strawberries. Then, I remind myself of the drug-fuelled psychedelic and surrealist nature of the song and the times that the song was written in but do take some solace from the idea of 'nothing is real' and yet very real and meaningful in many ways. At the time of writing the song, the location of Strawberry Fields belonged to a Salvation Army children's home where Lennon would go and play, and the song reflected his feelings of always feeling different in life compared to others. If you go there now, it is not just a tourist attraction, but it is an affluent area where everything is neat and tidy and a far cry away from the less affluent areas of Liverpool.

When I visited this place of surrealism as I know it from the song, I chatted with my son about the Beatles and their songs and I put some context of the times to the songs, and where they came from and why they were famous. I also talked about Martin Luther King and Malcolm X and how disabled people, gay people, black people amongst other groups were fighting for their rights, and with much of this time dominated by the Vietnam War. We also discussed going back to my father's town in Wales, and how our ancestors would have fought for their rights to vote in the Blaenavon Riot of 1868, following the more famous protests for votes like the Chartists in the Newport Rising nearby in 1839 and when workers in Merthyr Tydfil in 1831 raised a red flag, which socialists and revolutionaries followed suit in other revolutions in the world thereafter, where maybe our ancestors were involved with that too. We spoke about Alexander Cordell's novel, 'Rape of the Fair Country' (1959), that was loosely based on Blaenavon and where he wrote about Welsh people fighting for rights, justice, and survival, and that Welsh people and many others in many other places are still doing so today – challenging the often-unsaid effects of permanent colonialisation. I explained to him what life was like in the 1960s when his grandad was about the same age as the Beatles and how life was different and how their grandparents would have viewed the world, mostly Victorians and their attitudes to life, but how it still effects the idea and ways of life of my dad's generation. We often reflect on the fact that my grandfather was born in 1897 in Victorian times, my dad and I were born in 1946 and 1983 and my son in 2012, meaning that we cover three centuries between all four of us, and in child-friendly terms, discussed the historical, cultural, social, and political consequences of these time periods. It turned out to be an almighty reflective week with the passing of my dad, his grandad, and it felt like all that was real had become 'nothing is real'.

Could the same be said about psychology, is it real? I do not say that to be daft about whether it is real or not because I am a psychologist, I talk about psychology, I teach about psychology, and I know many psychologists – it must be real. But then again, for marginalised people, it is not real to them because of the repetitive themes and issues I have raised in this book. That is psychology, in all its forms, is not something that marginalised people connect with in a way that psychology can be transformative in their lives, so that they can live a happier, empowering, and inclusive life where their identities are completely accepted. The essence of this idea on whether psychology as we think we have known it is relevant in the 21st century for marginalised people will be explored in this chapter, through the lens of a queerying and imaginative 'posthuman community psychology'. Poulos (2006:113) suggested that even stories in our dreams should be a part of the ethnographic palette because dreams 'can cut through all the hubbub and haze and shadowy ambiguity of everyday life' (also see Richards, 2014a). This is what this chapter is about because I am just trying to imagine what psychology could look like through the haze and shadows and thinking about oneself and the intersectional factors that influence who we are and helped me to develop a critical consciousness and awareness of what psychology could become.

What is evident for me as a person, academic, researcher, and critical community psychologist is that psychology is flawed in many ways, but as many possibilities and hopes too that could make a genuine difference in people's lives, but how does psychology as whole begin to change and to revise what it can become that helps everyone. I posited earlier in the book that some of the ideas and perspectives that have emerged from critical/posthumanism might provide some revitalising and creative insights into what a future psychology could be. Could psychology become a psychology for all things and learn from values and principles set out by critical/community psychologists whilst taking both mainstream and critical/community psychology to another place that fits with the ways, purposes, and intersubjective lives of all that make up our communities.

This chapter will reflect on some ideas that explore some possibilities with a critical posthumanities edge in creating a 'posthuman community psychology' as a working title, where I wonder and wander through thoughts that have been influenced and intersected at micro and macro levels. The ideas will be influenced by some of the discussions I have presented in this book and will be influenced directly and indirectly around my experiences of working in the community, working with psychologists and other professionals, personal experiences, and debates with students. I do not present this chapter as a visionary or prophet even if the tone feels that way, but we must allow ourselves excuses and moments to be able to wonder and wander about psychology and have hopes about what psychology can become. In turn, psychology could be something that is genuinely useful and life-changing in a positive way for all, after all, all forms of psychology are not doing enough to become the kind of psychology that is suitable for marginalised people.

No more 'psychology'

Wonder

I am wondering what it would be like if psychology as we know it did not exist. No more labs, one-way mirror screens, cold rooms with basic furniture, eye-tracker equipment, snobbery, judgements, patriarchy, binaries, experiments, statistics, interviews, questionnaires, and psychology departments at universities.

I am wondering what it would be like if critical psychologists smiled for once in a while, were realist and helpful in changing the world. I am wondering if it is too easy to be critical, too easy to point the finger to say, 'you are wrong'.

Wander

I am wandering down the canal nearby and see new ducklings swimming in line with their mummy duck with the daddy duck watching from a distance. I see the dopey wood pigeons in the tree, bluffing their feathers, whilst the seagulls, black birds, and robins circle around for food and play with each other in their little families and partnerships. It makes me think of human babies and children, connecting with the world with an open mind, wondering and wandering what a magical world it can be and what there is to explore.

I then wander down the other end of the canal and see that a cat has butchered a duck and the family of ducks squawk and flap their wings and then fly away from their home with the ducks that remain. I see that the wood pigeons have been attacked by the angry family of crows and that the robins do not come into the garden anymore because the owner has stopped putting bird seed outside. I then put on the news on television and see that some babies have been abused and killed by their carers, relating to drugs and alcohol, and I wonder and wander about why some people never get to feel and see the magic of life like I do.

My wanderings here present a binary of good and bad, and we see this in psychology, science, and day-to-day life every day. This could be seen as psychology vs. other psychologies or good nature vs. bad nature, positive human experiences vs. negative human experiences. This is how psychologists, scientists, healthcare professionals, and people in general try to make sense of the world by distinguishing between ideas, concepts, behaviours, and identities, by placing it all into categories or distinctive groups, with little room for grey areas, overlaps, and pluralities. But I wonder if we stopped psychologising, being psychological or using the word 'psychology' or be able to redefine these words, would the world be a different place, for the better? Can we envision a future where there is no more 'psychology'?

This seems like a crazy idea, the idea of no more psychology and psychologising, but there is nothing wrong with trying to imagine a world without psychology as we know it. I have used the word 'psychology' throughout because that is a focal point to this book, and without using the word, readers would not know what I am referring to. To then talk about a 'posthuman community psychology' and use the word 'psychology' and then say 'let's not use the word' seems strange, however, my point is that what people understand psychology to be, from a biomedical, scientific stance, then it is the wrong place to start and so arguably the word 'psychology' is a barrier for change and different ways to think about what a 'human' is and what the study of behaviour should be. It is not enough to have more and more psychologies emerging as a way to challenge the traditional hold that contemporary psychology encompasses because psychology just becomes one giant snowball of problems in understanding the world. We need to rethink what this word means and consider a revolutionary change if psychology has a chance of adapting with the ever-changing world and humanhood, for it to be a psychology for the people.

Earlier in the book, I explored some of the positives of mainstream psychology that has been underpinned by billions of pounds where there is evidence that psychological interventions have reduced mortality, improved care, and impacted on policy and legislation. There have been in-roads to working across disciplines and qualitative research and this has been amalgamated into that that has helped to promote equality and inclusion. This is all positive and should be taken seriously, but the principles, values, methods, and philosophical perspectives of psychologists, neuroscientists, and psychiatrists are rooted in reductionist and logical empiricist ways of 'doing psychology', and this brings in money, power, and influence in ways that alienate marginalised groups and squeeze out more full on qualitative, creative, innovative methods that arguably are more likely to promote the voices of marginalised people. Whilst 'psychology' does a lot of good, it also does a lot of bad, and that bad is smoke screened by its success of bringing in billions of pounds and strengthening its scientific base with collaborators across the world and across disciplines. What would mainstream psychology look like if there was a decentring of science and empirical logicism, with marginalised groups at the heart of the power and decision-making? Well, it would probably not mean billions of pounds or world leading status because it would not be deemed scientific enough, so why would it change. Could 'psychology' be more powerful by working alongside and promoting the voices of the marginalised, or is 'psychology' the problem and the barrier?

It seems to me that we need to reconsider what psychology really is for people, and in all its diversities, positionalities, and identities, and it might be helpful to go beyond what we believe and know psychology to be to begin to do that. From a critical posthumanities perspective, humans have changed and keep changing. In fact, humans are always changing, and so it is not a surprise that humans are complex in complex surroundings and systems that change themselves, so for psychology to remain static in its scientific visions and methods, whilst with established big successes, it is not as successful for marginalised people. Although there might be lots of different types of psychologies that demonstrate the diversity of psychology and people, the fundamentals of what mainstream psychology is, is ever present and non-changing, ensuring that psychology fails to revolutionise the dark lives that many people face, yet it has the power to make a bigger difference than what it does. Maybe mainstream psychology in its current format needs people to be marginalised and excluded so it can continue to label, stereotype, marginalise, and exclude people, to help it bring in the huge funds. By doing so, it does not relinquish any power or control over people, ensuring that mainstream psychology is not fit for purpose for most people in its current form.

Mainstream psychology maintains big successes of power, money, and control, but it is an identity crisis, and it has always undergone an identity crisis with the shifting and changing approaches and waves over the course of the past 150 years, and yet, it remains the same somehow, in the way capitalism remains the same. I see similarities with mainstream and critical community psychology perspectives too, where the same kind of people who are rich, powerful, white, heterosexual, and educated doing the same things, saying the same things. I fit the same description and here I am proposing ideas for another 'psychology' too, so it seems to me that psychology cannot be and never has been what we think it to be, and our perception of it and how it is presented, organised, and controlled, remains embedded in empirical logicism, which is alien and exclusionary for most beings. This prevents raising direct questions, albeit it does in many ways, about what it means to be human. The very study of psychology concerns the 'mind' and 'behaviour' of people, but how can this be considered through entrenched, immoveable empiricist ideas and methods, whilst rejecting other ideas and methods. Mainstream psychology's positionality ensures that more and more questions can be raised about what it means to be human and about equalities for marginalised people who cannot meet the 'ideal' human underpinned by social, political cultural, and historic influences. For example, the principles that underpin humanistic psychology and indeed the influences this has had on critical/community psychology of all kinds, have ensured that traditional understandings of 'human' have been closed off and self-contained. This ensures established binaries between genders, races, disabilities, and other identities continue to be stuck and remain distant from the ideas around humans being ambiguous and multiple that a critical posthuman perspective can bring decentring people to a less privileged place above or under other people (see Massumi, 1992; Gibson, 2006; Gibson et al., 2021). Deleuze and Guattari's (1987) idea of 'assemblages' is useful because a recognition that something is constantly changing, and reinterpreting suggests that there is a constant shift between the connectivities between all things. All things are dynamic, intersect, and reconfigure, and this helps to understand what we are 'becoming'. Psychology is in this strange position of always being in a state of 'becoming' with the many psychologies that exist, and yet somehow, stays the same, pinned down by ideals that are not in line with what life and people are becoming.

I pointed out in Chapter 1 that the ontology of 'becoming' concerns leaning away from being fixed, and through assemblages, the process of becoming may be and influenced by many factors (see Fox & Alldred, 2017), meaning that becoming is a form of progression that intersects and is not linear and can break away or redirect itself whilst resisting set boundaries. Psychology changes, but never changes, and yet people and the world are forever in flux, which suggests that psychology as we know it cannot exist and is not fit for purpose in representing the intersubjectivities and diverse identities that we experience all the time. Therefore, psychology needs to redefine and reposition itself into something that resonates with a new materialistic position that sees living things as being in a world that is relational, plural, and uneven and cuts across dualistic dichotomies and boundaries. This new-materialist ontology, which is not in line with human universalism, ensures psychology can move towards a diversity and multiplicity that goes beyond the established dichotomies that were established a long time ago. In line with Herbrechter's perspective, a new paradigm of critical posthumanities thinking is emerging that does not just continue to challenge what 'human' means, it also considers the ever-changing contexts that living things reside in that are influenced by global challenges such as war, pandemics and continued environmental problems that earth is facing, alongside the ever more powerful digitalisation of life and biomedia, and the continued blurring's of relationships between non–human and human life forms. Psychology is at the heart of this but does not seem to realise it yet and yet the Anthropocene and biopolitics continues to be deconstructed and is becoming increasingly informed by strengthening processes in bioart, new media, and digital post/humanities. This theoretical foundation therefore analyses how people have shaped their lifestyles in line with digitalisation and virtual reality, alongside the conflicting traditions relating to the establishment of humanism, that can provide insights into what we might become or are becoming and how psychology can link with this and what it can become.

The word 'psychology', and we associate psychology within terms of its ideas, practices, and methods, is a barrier to opening up to different ideas, perspectives, and identities. Traditional definitions of psychology permeate across the world as a pathologising, psychologising, and medicalising force, which is not what psychology is to many or can be for marginalised people. For a posthuman community psychology future to take place, a brave leap of faith is needed to turn away from psychology and for that to be replaced not with a definitive other word, but with something that is meaningful, relational, exploratory, and contextual that embraces multiple assemblages. What do we have to lose by not just 'giving psychology away', but turning psychology upside down and shaking it about? The 'posthuman' cannot define the newer human condition and instead offers a spectrum on how we can understand power, identity, and all discourses. Therefore, a posthuman community psychology cannot be 'psychology', but psychology was never what we think it is anyway. Let us then begin with 'psychology', but like with the study of disabilities, do not end with psychology (see Goodley, 2011, 2013).

A becoming companion species – Cosmopolitan of life

Wonder

I am wondering what would become of our lives if we lived in peace and cared for one another, a common purpose, an acknowledgement that all things need one another.

Wander

I wander through some of my psychology books and roam through the pages thinking about the main approaches in mainstream psychology and what the critics have to offer. If we turned what we understand to be 'psychology' upside down from being a separated community of thinkers and practitioners, and turned towards a community of practices, where divisions between professionals and marginalised people were no longer there, we would understand the world and people more than what we do now. We have seen dogs with their owners in restaurants and public houses, we have known people able to have babies through the magic of science, a people's creation, and we have seen how we can communicate with astronauts in space and put robots on planets. We have seen the power of communities when people come together in wars, and the power of voices through protests and social movements through past and recent history.

I imagine myself in a Marvel film and think is this what a future cosmopolitan life could be, humans with magic powers, flying from one planet to another, coming back to save earth occasionally, if earth still exists during these climate changes? Will terminators take over the planet? Will the dinosaurs return? Will Jesus finally walk down from Heaven and take us to a place of pure whiteness with everyone singing hymns and arias forever? Can psychology be bold, imaginative, and go to places that people have not gone before?

To turn 'psychology' upside down and rethink what 'psychology' can become also raises questions about day-to-day life and communities and what we might become as individuals. Through history and our analysis of history, and this is usually from a white man's gaze ensuring a narrow and linear view of life, we have looked for an afterlife or a future that is better than the past, and we may take comfort from this or become depressed at the realisation that the afterlife is not what it might end up being or the future is necessarily any better than the past. The main approaches in psychology have set out how humans should think, feel, and behave, or this is how humans think, feel, and behave, within rigid structures of thinking, not fully recognising the significance we all play in all our communities and with each other and as individuals.

This makes me think about the importance of connection, being relational and part of something beyond the specific little worlds we live in. A 'cosmopolitan of life' (Nayar, 2014) recognises that we all need each other, with new ideas, new visions and new connections, and a reductionist and scientific psychology alone cannot provide that, nor can communities change and take action without the right tools, expertise, and approaches that mainstream psychology has to offer. What could a 'becoming companion of species' mean in the context of psychology? I find it difficult to visualise or comprehend, but in Chapter 1, I examined Nayar's (2014) ideas around the human co-evolving and sharing everything from ecosystems to life processes of all kinds and how technology is a part of human identities. This perspective in a time of technological and biomedical developments is useful for psychologists because of the psychological aspects of these advancements, changes, and ideological positions, which helps to reimage established humanistic perceptions and the politics that sets out humans from other forms of life as exclusionary.

The idea of 'co-evolvement' opposed to 'survival of the fittest' acknowledges that we are all symbiotic with all things and therefore we must become aware, embrace, and develop through interconnections and mergers with all life forms and be open-minded about our 'human' existence as being much more than we have known it to be. Nayar's 'companion species' that is becoming and something that becomes a way of life to form a multispecies citizenship implies that we must think about life and humanhood in different ways and from Nayar's perspective, because technological changes have ensured that. A cynic might say that the points I am making here might suggest that we start to release animals from zoos and let tigers live amongst us or in the spirt of community, maybe invite a lion around for dinner with their cubs. I am not saying that, and maybe the point is focused on how we all need each other through the big issues such as global climate change. Animals and other life forms are changing and dying because of climate change, and we know that the many marginalised groups are losing their islands, their homes, their identities because of climate change, almost always in the poorest areas in the world, but this is happening in rich places too. I would love to say that critical/community psychology has been at the forefront of these issues, yet critical/community psychology has only just touched the surface in the past ten years (Riemer & Reich, 2011). At the heart of critical/community psychology is the ecological theory or metaphor, and so to ignore the magnitude of climate changes and its effects will be a travesty for the most marginalised and all of us. Critical/community psychology and global climate change are strongly linked to values like social justice and wellbeing, and yet have not combined well together, but then the mainstream psychology analysis of climate change generally looks for relationships and patterns of individual behaviour relating to aggression, violence, and conflict, so neither forms of psychology have been at the forefront of actual change and difference (see Miles-Novelo & Anderson, 2019). This could be because of the issues I have raised in this book, and maybe psychology is due a rethink about how psychology and its resources, expertise, skills, and influences, and how it can become within communities, and how it can tackle a world issue like climate change means that there is much that we could be positive about through collaboration.

A 'becoming companion species' as a cosmopolitan way of life links in with the idea of a 'posthuman citizenship', so our co-evolution with other life forms ensures that from a biological and biometric point of view, our bodies are changing, and our brains are always changing. Therefore, how we do psychology and how we think about humans also needs to change, in line with how our world is changing too. The human can be considered to be a 'node' that embraces a citizenship that is embodied and interconnects with the environment (Nayar, 2014). This means that we are not objective organisms or a laboratory's plaything and that we can only understand people, living things, and our communities or one whole community through the intersectional connections that can only be understood in context with how we interact with our world, technologies, and biology (some might say this is my own reductionist and hypocritical view of psychology), but if there was a companion species that is always becoming, and this develops more understanding and care for each other, then there might just be less discriminatory and exclusionary practices, and acceptance that an accompaniment way of life is needed for real survival and happiness.

In Chapter 2, I briefly discussed the idea that for a becoming companion of species to emerge, the multiple stands of psychology would need to be a collective rather than sold as different psychologies that often work in separation, and are rivals, with limited work between, for example, say clinical and critical psychologists or forensic and critical/community psychologists. Why should there be that division when all kinds of psychologies and psychologists have much to offer one another and their participants and community members. By changing that dynamic to something that is becoming, a new identity for psychology could develop that embraces both the individual and individual in context and other life forms. This links in with principles of critical community psychology set out by Kagan et al. (2021) such as diversity, innovation, liberation, commitment, critical reflection, and humility, but a becoming companion of species can also be influenced and revitalised with the strengths and positives that mainstream psychology can provide too. Mainstream psychology has demonstrated that it can bring in money to advance research that has the potential to change people's lives for the better. It has also demonstrated that it can help to reduce mortality, improve the quality of life, and having impact on policy and legislation in all areas of day-to-day life and within major societal institutions at local, national, and international levels. This lends itself potentially well to a companion of species with all forms of mainstream, critical, and community psychologies, using a range of methods and skills across multiple disciplines and professions, ensuring that the political is still at the heart of the cosmopolitan.

Some readers will think this is fantastical and delusional, the idea that all forms of 'psychology' can somehow come together to form a new kind of 'discipline' or life form, and indeed, that would mean working across many other disciplines, professions, and professionals a psychologist might not ordinarily work with. Maybe psychology is just too diverse and too entrenched in its ways to adapt and why adapt if it ensures that people have successful careers, it brings in big money and continues to be a popular subject to study, regardless of what it represents. Yet, psychology is a bizarre contradiction of engaging in new technology, new ideas, and innovations and this can be seen in many publications and practices, and yet somehow still be handcuffed to principles of empiricism that do not connect with marginalised people, who are mostly the subjects of experiments and science. Whilst established therapies like cognitive behavioural therapy have helped people and would indicate that sometimes a linear and simplistic approach to helping people is a success, the idea of a becoming companion species though is about how we can all work together and go beyond the boundaries in place around psychology that does not place blame and 'the problem' on individuals. A becoming companion species can be about those principles set out by Kagan et al. (2021), but they can also be about everything else if psychologists really tried to go beyond their own boundaries. A 'companion of species' would appreciate and intersect through biology, technology, as well as political, cultural, social, and discursive influences that make up our multiple identities. But this has always happened for people and the world, in psychology, however, this has been reduced in a way that ensures we become what psychology and its partners in science and medicine want us to become, which is counterproductive and driven by neoliberal principles in the main, ensuring fewer people benefit. A way of becoming must be mutually beneficial, with all living things, and this critical posthumanities outlook would help psychology become a space for accompaniment to flourish.

A becoming companion species that links in with what psychology can offer can be inclusive, feminist, queer, scientific, technological, earth, and cosmos and this inter-trans-approach can overcome the status quo of 'Royal Science' and 'cognitive capitalism' that encapsulates 21st century psychology through its power of media and culture, financialisation, and bio-genetic and technological advanced capitalism (Braidotti, 2017). We are humans who are becoming, and always are becoming, new people, and 'psychology' needs to be new for a new people and not stuck on aged ideas of false hopes. The psychology as we know it can be a part of something more powerful (powerful in an empowering way) for all things rather than remain in its own bubble of science and false hopes of what it claims to do for people. Psychology, for all its expertise, practices, applications, and insights, could be part of a revolution that connects with all things and be a force for good where people can be happier and connected but radicalised in a way that does not scare people. A becoming psychology can go beyond the boundaries of positive psychology and self-help books of person-centredness and focus more on believing in one another and that we all have something to offer, which links in with values that are well established in critical community psychology, but values that underpin the work of many mainstream psychologists and community psychologists.

Assemblage approach to care and community

Wonder

I wonder about why person-centredness for many people is abuse, powerlessness and exclusionary and not what it sets out to be

Wander

I wander about in a care home where they care for older adults with disabilities. There is a hot large room that feels stuffy, with wiffs of lavender and rose water, somehow mixed in with a bit of bleach in the air and I see several people spread out in individual chairs in a horseshoe shape. I imagine if my dad was still alive and what it would have been like to have seen him in one of these places, the same places he had spent years working in, caring for people with humour, kindness, and humility, and it makes me question why so much abuse and neglect happens in these prisons for older people with disabilities.

I think about what happens to the man who likes to put on dresses, paint his nails and put on his high heels, especially the clothes with silver sequins and bits of glitter.

I think about the bisexual woman who wants to play with a woman she wants to woo but is not allowed to chat her up because she is stuck in her chair and needs to wait for someone to take her over.

I think about the trans man who gets ignored and is left until last before they can have their turn to have a wash.

I think about the carers, staff, business owners, and officials who run these places and think about how they have similar identities, similar values, have the skills to care and encourage, be creative, share expertise, and experiences and skills. But somehow, do not always seem to care, forget how similar they are to the people they are offering care to, forget their common values and forget how to use their skills to be creative, innovative, caring, and empowering for the people who do not want to forget or stop being who they are.

Earlier, I reflected on some critical posthuman ideas and about how it could relate to a rethinking of what understand to be psychology, and how it could become a part of a companion of species, and I questioned psychology's very existence and worth to people, in a world, a cosmos, that is always changing. Whilst that would be part of a cosmopolitan that allows difference and Other to be what they want to be without prejudice, difference does bring division, with different expectations and norms, but it also means that for care and support and help one might need. This is currently viewed from a 'person-centredness' and 'care in the community' perspective in the West, which in my view cannot work and does not work, as effectively as policy, theorists and practitioners like to postulate. For a companion species that is becoming, the voices of the most marginalised need to be genuine power-brokers, in collaboration with others, to decide what care and communities should be like and become a space where happiness, respect, and love is at the heart of this, which means an assemblage approach to care within a companion species is needed. This means looking beyond the out-of-date person-centred approaches that are inconsistent with helping marginalised people, and instead a focus is needed on turning this upside down into something that is accepting of difference. And recognises the complexities of care and support for community members that is transformative and inclusive and not tied into neoliberal and capitalist ideologies of costs, outcomes, and 'evidence-based' initiatives that are top-down and disempowering. We all need help, we all need care, in some form or another, at some point, and for many, this is needed all the time, and this is not going to change even with a becoming way of life to come.

My reflections in my wonderings and wanderings highlight the challenges that come with caring for people, often in controlled and disempowering environments. But this can be seen in many walks of life and within 'caring' professions where there is a mish mash of complicated power relations, diversities, multiple identities, and yet a 'person-centred approach' is this idea that all people will be cared for and respected. This ensures that identities are stifled, excluded, and it places people at different levels of power, rubber-stamped by being 'person-centred'. If one of the premises of this book is to say that what we understand to be human is not as it really is, then how we care for people, in a potential becoming companion species also needs to be turned upside down. What could an assemblage approach to care and community mean?

I have reflected on the idea of 'psychology in the community', and for me is not as positive as it sounds. For instance, much of the work that is done in the name of 'community psychology' has strong parallels with mainstream psychology, so the methods and ideas that underpin psychology are taken into the community. However, it is often without any real emphasis on being participatory and making decisions with community members and marginalised groups, ensuring that top-down approaches encapsulate much of what is published in critical/community psychology. Even though one of the main differences for community psychologists from mainstream psychology is to see people in context, there is a failure to engage at the intersubjective levels of experience with marginalised people, and this is counterproductive because the skills, roles, and expertise that can contribute to change in their lives could make a big difference. If a person-centred approach is meant to develop a genuine connection between psychologists and other care professionals with marginalised groups and individuals, then why do people face abuse and have disempowering experiences? I have previously discussed this issue in Chapter 4, and it is worth reiterating that people are expected to be 'person-centred' and apply a 'person-centred approach' in many professionals, not just psychologists, but it has become meaningless and counter-intuitive in people wanting to be who they are and what they want to become. The reality is that the 'person-centred approaches' we are familiar with are underpinned by biomedical approaches, which continue to ensure that voices are not heard, and choice is taken away and 'treatments' are based on bio-medical interventions and basic psychological interventions. Cure and ameliorative interventions are the order of the day, and this diminishes voices, inclusivity, and stifles the many identities that encapsulates a person. The congruent relationships that are meant to be at the heart of person-centred approaches do not exist for many, ensuring that person-centred approaches only help people to an extent.

An assemblage approach to care and community therefore would not just be about making sure older people in care homes have their bums wiped (this is important) or that they have more variety in their dinners every day, or if an autistic person wants to shout and swear because that is how they are feeling rather than being pinned down and controlled like they are a violent person. Instead, an 'assemblage approach' would prioritise understanding that through assemblages we are influenced by many factors, and we need to be cared for with those changes, differences, and becomings at the heart of how we care, because we are too ambiguous and do not live well within set and clear-cut humanised boundaries. Tokenistic decisions relating to including the person in their care, which is enshrined in lots of recent policy around care is ameliorative at best. People who need care, and that is all of us at some point in some way, should be at the very heart of decision-making at all levels, but in a way that does not lead to a new policy that encompasses everyone, another good sounding policy, but policies that are fluid and moveable to genuinely ensure that all identities and marginalised groups of people are really empowered and are happier. This would be a shift from the medicalised underpinnings to health and social care and person-centredness that are driven by pathological, positivist, and reductive understandings of the body and mind. This would not work within a posthuman community psychology way of becoming and does not work now for many, meaning an intercon nected approach to care is needed that is intersectional, queer, discursive, and relational. The well-intentioned meanings of the humanistic psychology that emerged with Rogers and others lost meaning a long time ago, and its application is complicated and maybe does not consistently fulfil the role of empowering people as much as we convince ourselves.

Multiple methods, approaches, and tools – Relational applications

---

Wonder

I wonder what it would be like if ethically approved psychological experiments that have been applied to people with the label of autism were instead created and facilitated by the same people.

Wander

I wander about a psychology department at a university and see all the technical equipment, laboratories, the one-way mirrors, the state-of-the-art technology that is used to detect whether you are telling lies or not and notice the small rooms for interviews.

I wander past these areas and look at the technology and think about what it would be like if those people of all ages, genders, ethnicities, and other demographics used this technology and used the technology to explore their own identities and behaviour and worked in collaboration with mainstream psychologists to use the technology to explore disabilities, ASD, and all the other labels in the DSM. Would we find out more about who we are and what we can become?

I have scribbled down some ideas on what it would be like to take the unthinkable leap into the unknown by suggesting that psychology as we know it should be refashioned and reworked because it is not fit for purpose as a static and entrenched way of understanding the mind, behaviour, and context. I have also vaguely considered what could replace that in part with the idea of a becoming companion species and that aspects of psychology could play a genuine and important part in that development. Also, how some of the ideas that influence that might help us to think beyond the simplicities of person-centred care and approaches, but how can we do this and what is at our disposal to make changes happen, make a difference. For example, could the methods, approaches, and tools that are available and will become available in the future help marginalised people to create their cartographies that provide more insights, on an equal level, into what makes us who we are and our place in the world. Does the dancing and playing of children in a playground, carefree, or someone singing to themselves happily with their air pods on, a better way of knowing people, with what they use in those moments to express themselves? What is for sure is that more methods, tools, and technologies are available to us that allow us to express and become identities that humans might not have been before, suggesting that we are very much in a posthuman period, but psychology despite having the technology, methods, and influences at its disposal, is still stuck in old-fashioned ways that are not as becoming. Nonetheless, mainstream and critical community psychology are not a lot different. Yes, there are lots of studies where researchers have used methods and tools that you would not think about in mainstream psychological contexts of research such as poetry, dance, music, arts, storytelling through creative means, and varieties of visual methods such as photovoice and the use of apps, but much more could be done, especially on a digital technology front.

In this context, Condie and Richards (2022) discussed some ideas around the relationship between critical/community psychology and digital technology. First, to be able to think about this, we used a digital autoethnography to discuss the ideas and the paper we put together. Whilst this is not entirely new, after all, many would have done something similar during the Covid-19 pandemic, this method highlighted the relational and how you make use of what you have available at your disposal rather than defined methods where you must follow instructions. Some of the ideas that emerged helped us to think about what a future critical/community psychology might look like from a 'digital' perspective, and we boldly called out that a new 'digital community psychology' would add value. Just writing a paper via email demonstrated that as psychologists there needs to be a flexibility and open-mindedness about how to connect with one another, whether it be traditional or non-traditional communicative methods. However, the main point we wanted to make was that although psychology has embraced the 'digital' and on a small scale, critical/community psychology has done the same, there are clear issues, and it is the same old issues that encapsulate contemporary psychology. For example, we pointed out that mainstream psychology has used digital tools to manipulate, persuade, and harm and those digital products are in themselves psychologised to interpret and effect our behaviours that control what we do. You can think about this in terms of downloading items or games or how we manipulate pictures, a form of 'persuasive design' (Brennan, 2020), ensuring that there are big ethical questions that psychology has not ever addressed. In addition, digital data and its use is in line with the experimental and positivist ways of psychology, and this datafication of society fits well with quantitative approaches to understanding behaviour, and this can be seen across society in government, private corporations, and established institutions such as in the education system. Therefore, a digital psychology that encompasses a form of activism links in well with many of the values of all kinds of community psychology and could be disseminated within mainstream psychology to help bring people together, with a view that it is together, not to gain in the capitalist sense. A posthuman and new-materialist perspective on how we understand and use technology can bridge the gap between societal levels and local community levels, making it relational and inter-connected, where change can take place when needed to challenge social justice issues.

In Chapter 1, I suggested that in relation to digital technology many millions of people might not have access or the means to be able to use digital technology. Indeed, for some marginalised groups like prisoners or people who are sectioned, they might not be allowed to use digital technology, but that does not mean that digital technology is not influencing those people or controlling people and therefore everyone needs to be involved and are involved. Similarly, the many creative and visual methods that are available are contributing to our understanding of who we are and how our world is taking shape. This can be seen in social media at an individual level and every so often at a greater level, we hear about a new telescope that can see worlds billions of light years away. The technology itself is symbolic of the changing nature of humans at the intersectional and intersubjective level and that we are part of a something much greater that is relevant to all living things.

A posthuman community psychology that intersects and is open to all perspectives about how we might think about humans and psychology and communities needs to be able to explore and interrogate and engage with tools and ideas that can lead to us becoming. The ideas in the book would suggest that any method works, if it works for someone and the people around them. So, if that means methods of engagement are scientific in nature, traditional methods such as experiments, random controlled trials, or more creative from art and craft to dance, then so be it, if it means there is a level playing field between people when engaging with such methods. The cynic would say this is about people 'dancing around the maypole' and making daisy chains in the meadows, but in fact, it is saying that as relational beings that are forever in flux, then whatever suits people, whatever makes people feel happy and feel connected is what counts, and our understanding of humans, behaviours, the mind, and contexts might be better understood.

Decolonising and deideologising companionships

Wonder

I wonder what it would be like if psychology of all kinds was mostly made up of a diverse set of people including, all ethnicities, all nations, all sexualities, all genders, and all ages amongst other marginalised groups and identities in our world.

Wander

I wander back through the psychology curriculums that were indoctri-
nated into me all those years ago at university and I think how similar
it is for the curriculums that children experience in schools – white
people in pictures and photographs, histories of the world from a white
perspective, almost entirely heterosexual and gendered, delivered by
mostly those same people in those books, worksheets, and activities. I
wander through the education I have known and think about what this
all means for marginalised people but think about what a difference
psychology could bring to the world if it was brave enough to decolonise and deideologise.

Psychology as we know it cannot stay the same if humans and the world
is always changing, as societies and communities are always changing, and
earth and the universe itself is always changing. One of the significant reasons why psychology needs to change and must change because it needs to be
decolonised and deideologise itself and move to a place that engages with all
people on an equal level. Whilst decoloniality is being explored more than
ever, and all forms of psychology are being challenged to decolonise itself,
this has been a very slow process, and psychology remains the old-fashioned
structure that it is, and any real change is likely to be slow. A becoming
companion species that might benefit from aspects of what we have understood psychology to be could not emerge if the psychological continues to
be colonial and driven by traditional ideologies of how we must view the
world. Fanon's work on highlighting the political and power in psychology
epitomises the need to explore the intersubjective experiences of everyday
life for marginalised people to ensure a progressive and inclusive politics can
emerge. This has infiltrated the works of more recent writers of decoloniality in community psychology circles (see Chapter 4), where there are calls
to reclaim and reimage ways of being and promote marginalised voices by
centring their concerns by the subtle and more blatant effects of colonialism.
Psychology, empirical logicism, and science in general are very much part of
a system that is white dominated and underpinned by capitalist and neoliberal
principles ensuring that the status quo remains, which is dominated by the
same identities now as they were hundreds of years ago. Authors who write
about decoloniality and psychology/community psychology seek to transform and centralise forgotten voices and to re-understand the entrenched
Western interpretations of people's experiences, norms, and values to a position where people can speak freely about who they are, how they feel, in their
contexts (Sonn et al., 2022a).

This helps me to queery my work in the community and reminds me
of the Freirean influences on my work. A key concept of Freirean ideas is

'consciousness' or 'critical consciousness' that goes some way in helping to radically transform people and communities by becoming more aware of their contexts and to seek engaged participation to find solutions and make changes. Through conscientisation, we can rethink our world and maybe see it more for what it is, in a way that was unimaginable before. Whilst Freire did not develop his work at a time when there was the Internet or social media or other forms of digital technology where many can access information and ideas to make them aware of something at the click of a finger, meaning that awareness is arguably more powerful and likely than before, the new knowledge one gains of their present realities, provides the basis to make changes. This is not possible for some because of extreme poverty or homelessness, so the means to use this technology is not possible, but the empowering effects of awareness and dialogue has the potential to challenge established institutes and powerbases like psychology, and by challenging psychology, there is hope it can be fit for purpose or reimagined as something that is becoming, liberating, decolonial, and deideologised.

Montero (2012) has also made some useful points that link in well with some of the ideas relating to critical posthumanities and Freirean thinking. For example, Montero points out that when we think about communities we think about its history, resources, who is in or who is out, boundaries relating to territory, and other things, but it is the 'relatedness' between people that is significant (influenced by Freirean principles). This can be virtual or physical at different times and places, and there is still this knowing between people and links well with the idea that 'being' relates to who we are connected with that we are all connected to. It does not stop us from being individuals, but we only become individuals in how relationships, constructions, and connections with the people around us and wider contexts, and this idea if implemented it is possible to reduce that binary with Other and reduce the exclusionary practices that come with being Other (also see Levinas, 1977/1995 in Montero, 2012). With mainstream psychology (in certain respects) and the different forms of critical/community psychology placing emphasis on inclusion, participation, and equality, with chippings of social justice values and practices seeping through, being able to relate to people is more likely to avoid exclusion and challenge abusive systematic power.

I then think about what decolonising and deideologising companionships could become? I think Freire and Fanon still have a place in helping us understand how genuine companionships of accompaniment can emerge that promotes the voices of marginalised people and ensuring that to understand people and life, we must understand the political to make real change. The idea of decolonialisation and deideologisation is not new and both concepts have been written about for decades and within and outside of psychology, but both are playing a more consistent role in writings and publications within critical/community psychology, and these ideas, visions, and challenges are needed for psychology to be of relevance to most humans. Posthuman community psychology would encompass a decolonised and deideologised way of becoming that is about accompaniment, relatedness, and awareness of the world around us, a dream that needs to be a reality to moves beyond the Eurocentric and Americanised gaze on humans and all beings, and instead we can gaze at each other and the world around us in new ways.

New ideas, new solutions – Beyond the 'psych' and within the 'psych' (across disciplines)

> **Wonder**
>
> I wonder about why psychologists are reluctant to reach out to other disciplines, perspectives, ideas – should we dare to go beyond the 'psychological'?
>
> **Wander**
>
> I wander down to the beach in Liverpool, UK, and I can see Wales across the water, and I think about posthumanism and robots and imagine Terminators marching down the promenade, and when I get that image out of my head, I think about existentialism and phenomenology and how I deliver philosophy to students in lectures. I think about what the social worker might say about safeguarding when I see a young child walking seemingly alone away from home, or a support worker when I see a man hiding in a box, homeless and drinking a can of beer at midday, on the edge of the boulders near the sea. I walk away from this beach of ideas and reflections about what different professionals, practitioners, and disciplines do for people and what they could do together.

Traditionally, mainstream psychology has sat alone somewhere, in-between the natural sciences and social sciences. In effect, mainstream psychology has always had an identity crisis, which could suggest that it is not fit for purpose or that it has always been in a state of flux in such a way that it never admits. However, psychology in all parts has adapted in certain respects and recognised that working across disciplines and methodologies adds value on many fronts. Yet, more needs to be done, after all, new ideas mean new solutions to the problems people face in communities and what we have learnt and developed under the title of 'psychology' can help people more extensively, and to do this in collaboration with other disciplines and go beyond the 'psych' can only be a good thing.

A posthuman community psychology that hopes to become and be relational can remain on the edges of 'contemporary' psychology. It goes without saying that like critical psychology and many forms of critical/community psychology, a posthuman community psychology needs to relate and embrace other disciplines, and not just disciplines that sounds like they fit like 'community development' or 'social work', but any discipline that adds something that helps change to occur or adds another philosophical angle to our thinkings. When I meet people, I have often been told that I am really a sociologist in disguise, or I should be a sociologist. Sometimes people have said community psychology does not exist or simply think I am a clinical psychologist, and I reflected on this in an earlier chapter. Nonetheless, each time, and often without saying it because I always feel it will take me a long time to explain (like this book), I think to myself, that is maybe why I am a critical community psychologist in the first place because the traditions that I come from (Kagan et al., 2021, 2022) embrace different disciplines, perspectives, and viewpoints, and a significant part of our work has been directly influenced by marginalised voices. So, the voices across the spectrum of disciplines, whatever they may be, can all add value in some way to thinking about a psychology that is becoming, and how we might view what a 'human' might be.

Justice for all, roles for all

Wonder

I wonder about what happened to that older woman who stole gravy in a retail shop I worked at 20 years ago.

Wander

I wander back to different examples of injustice that I have witnessed in community projects, day-to-day life, and just in the local area. I think about that older woman and how she was frog-marched from the gravy aisle to the front of the shop, as I stacked shelves, where the security guards were joyful at getting their 'catch of the day' and phoning the police, and I remember the face of the woman looking completely lost. The security guards never asked if she was ok, if she needed support, or whether she picked up the gravy by mistake because her mind was on other things.

This sense of injustice is maybe not the most obvious example of injustice compared to what we witness on the daily news or read about in books. It was just a small example of someone being treated in a way that was not right, but one that would have had negative connotations for that person has she was taken away in a police van with feelings of fear to go in shops again, a new mistrust of authorities, a re-emergence of mental health issues that might not have led to help and support, or fears of being labelled as a criminal and other things. I was only a teenager at the time and had no voice or influence that would have made a difference, yet for me, there was a sense of injustice that I still remember today, and I have seen the equivalent many times over before and since then.

In my introduction to the book and at the beginning of Chapter 1, I queeried some of the injustices I have faced relating to my identities, abuse, marginalisation in schools and the local community, and how this might have affected who I have become and continue to become. I also acknowledged that my privileged position and that I make mistakes and cause problems as well, and I think that sense of reflecting and musing helps me to be a more positive person and to cope in a way that others might not who have come from my background. Yet, this is easier said than done, and when reflecting on the lives of the people I have worked with in the communities and in workplaces, justice has not always prevailed and probably never will for many. Many of the young people I worked with who were homeless for instance felt that there was nothing to aspire to and that there was no role for them in their communities. They felt barriers were always in the way because of their race, gender, sexualities, age, and other intersectional factors. The education system suits some people over others, but so do workplaces, services, and institutions, ensuring that equal justice for all and roles for all is not possible in the current systems that we live in. Similarly, within psychology, there are only so many roles that can be filled, by specific and qualified people, but the power of the tradition psychologies like clinical and forensic is dominated by white, wealthy, and educated people, ensuring that psychology in its present form is a discipline for specific people, the same people who create the DSM or the ICD or hold societal power, run institutions, own big businesses, and banks. Mainstream psychology like much of society ensures that there cannot be justice for all and roles for all and this cognitive capitalism (see Braidotti, 2019) needs to be extinguished.

At the heart of a posthuman community psychology, where a becoming companion of species emerges, justice needs to be at the centre, where all voices count and that voices contribute to a becoming space where people feel wanted and cared for in a way that would be revolutionary for psychology and beyond. I have already discussed that decolonising of psychology is still needed and a deideologising of psychology is needed and this will help to ensure people are not excluded and get justice when they demand it, in the right possible ways. Psychologists and professionals, students, and others from other disciplines and beyond also can play a part in that role development, bringing in experiences and skills that might pave a way to a better chance for justice and inclusion.

Summary

Psychology, in all its forms, reminds me of a collage of messiness, complexity, and colours, something to gaze at and wonder about, which seems to resonate with a critical posthumanities outlook of relationality, multiplicity, and togetherness. However, at the same time, psychology is bizarrely strangulated by powerful scientific and medicalised underpinnings that prevent it from growing into something that becomes something that all people connect with and can contribute towards. Holding onto that thought, this chapter put forward some reflections on how one kind of a 'posthuman community psychology' might look. Reflecting on some of the points I have made means I can see that this kind of psychology is a becoming psychology that intersects across different psychologies, including mainstream and mainstream/critical community psychology, but with a view to not seeing these psychologies in isolation, and instead as part of something that can be greater. Most of the ideas and the analysis is not new and can be recognised in lots of work in the name of 'psychology', but that means we can play around with psychology and make it be whatever we want it to be, even if far-fetched – it is better than keeping with the status quo that ensures psychology continues to contribute to the seeming exclusion of marginalised people.

Critical posthuman perspectives are a useful way to rethink what all kinds of psychologist or psychologies can become because a common respect for all things, that being humans or other life forms, and for their 'fluid' identities, is a value that is underrated and often ignored by psychologists regardless of ethical guidelines and morality. Thinking about psychology with a critical posthuman analysis could help psychologists look beyond the hardened boundaries of science to think about the wider contexts more, going beyond the individual and embracing the evolving systems around us, where understanding human behaviour can be understood in the context of the human interaction with all life forms, technology, and biology. A collective psychology can intersect between individuals, contexts, and all things, and by doing so, a new identity emerges that is always in flux, ensuring that 'psychology' is a becoming assemblage that works equally with all beings. In addition, terming this chapter and book as 'posthuman community psychology' is not about a rebranded version of critical/community psychology or mainstream psychology, but it is about daring to intersect across psychology, of all kinds, to make use of resources, skills, and to share power and grow resilience as force for good in times that are always changing anyway. Psychologists can learn from other disciplines like critical disability studies because it unravels the politics of 'normality' and emphasises the need for mutuality and cooperation as opposed to competition and difference. A 'companion species' would mean an appreciation of biology, technology, cultural, political, social, historical, and multiple identities that make us who we are. Posthumanism rejects the binaries and autonomous subjectivity, and we are inclined to apply to our understanding of human behaviour. We should be respecting the multiple, diverse, and complex nature and nurture of what it means to be human and be able to seek to apply this within our spaces at every level. After all, the Eurocentric and American-centric basis of 'human' 'never was a universal or neutral term to begin with' (Braidotti, 2019:35), but a way of becoming is about how we might glide across the assemblages that disrupt the very entrenched binaries and definitions that define/or not define us in all our intersections. Psychology is already posthuman, and the barrier to accepting this is because the emphasis in psychology is on needing to be a 'science' and 'medical' to receive big funds, more power and more influence, therefore, the idea of redefining itself directly makes mainstream psychologists wobble and some psychologists will dismiss these ideas as something that is not 'psychology'. Yet, by accepting a posthuman turn that psychology has been going through over the decades arguably, it could ensure that psychology can become a better psychology that is fit for purpose for marginalised people.

Mainstream psychology and critical/community psychologies of all kinds need to come together and develop a 'psychology' that goes beyond fairy story values of 'goodness' and instead needs to look at the world around them and see the bigger picture. Critical/community psychologists reject mainstream psychology for many reasons and vice versa, but the reality is that they need one another and are related and have more in common than they like to admit, and by coming together with hope, building relationships in creative ways, we might then have a psychology for the people that can be a powerful force for good. Let us hear more about the lives and contexts from which psychologists have emerged and works and let us read their stories and accounts of life and let them connect with day-to-day people rather than hiding behind a one-way mirror, and psychology can become a psychology for all, a new posthuman community psychology.

6 Posthuman community psychology and disabled people – A reflection

For much of this book, I have constructed a narrative that has led up to the presentation of what a 'posthuman community psychology' might look like in Chapter 5, influenced by many things, including my personal, academic, and practice experiences of working in the community and influenced by my knowledge around psychology and critical/community psychology. Added to this, I have drawn on aspects of Braidotti, Nayar, and other posthuman thinkers' works encompassed within a 'critical posthumanities' framework, to reflect on what psychology is or never was and what it can become, particularly when working with marginalised people.

The difficulties of doing a book like this are that I am drawing on big themes and big ideas, and this ensures that the book is full of contradictions, hypocrisies, clumsy statements, and repetition, and so to reduce all this to a 'posthuman community psychology' is problematic and cumbersome. The ideas of what a 'posthuman community psychology' could look like to some readers will be that they are awkward and not realistic, and one that is based on one person's imagination, or even lack of it, but then again, when has psychology ever been straightforward? When has humanhood been easy to define and when have the marginalised stopped being marginalised? The book is about reflecting on my experiences of being a critical community psychologist, who like many other psychologists of all kinds, wants to see psychology be the best that it can be. One way to begin to do that is to try to think outside the box, be creative and imaginative, and try to be as real as you can be because if you cannot start to do that, then the status quo remains, which for marginalised people means continued exclusionary practices, hate crime, false labelling, disempowerment, and being voiceless.

Without doubt, postulating general and vague ideas of what a 'posthuman community psychology' could be needs to be scrutinised further, and for this chapter, I will try to do that by exploring what each idea that I explored in Chapter 5 could mean for disabled people. I am exploring this marginalised group because I have drawn on that group through the book and much of my ideas and work over the years are influenced by disciplines such as 'critical disability studies'. By considering disabled people in the context of a 'posthuman community psychology', the analysis to follow could also be relevant for

DOI: 10.4324/9781003057673-6

other marginalised groups too and intersects through different identities such as genders, ages, ethnicities, and sexualities.

No more 'psychology' as we know it – Is this what disabled people need?

In Chapter 5, I proposed the idea of not just redefining what 'psychology' is because of all its complexities, but I suggested that the word itself is no longer a fair and sensible way to think and label what we think psychology is in its current state and how we understand the ever-changing identity of 'human'. Whilst the idea will seem absurd for many readers, especially when I call myself a psychologist and have gained so much from what psychology is perceived to be, my experiences of working with marginalised groups would imply that this would be welcomed.

The use of the word 'psychology' in discussions relating to disability, which can be seen in the field of critical/disability studies and within the day-to-day practices of daily life and care for disabled people, is mostly considered to be pathological and individualising, and associated with psychologising and exclusionary practices for many disabled people (see Goodley & Lawthom, 2005a), and I do not see that changing anytime soon. For many disabled people, 'psychology' or the 'psychological' or 'psychologist' are dirty words because they are associated with control, misjudgement, labelling, and the consequences of labelling. This relates to mainstream psychology, but there has been hope with the developments of psychologies such as critical/community and critical psychology because they are viewed as psychologies that help to promote voices and challenge exclusionary and oppressive practices, ensuring that from that perspective, psychology is a political, cultural, social, historical, and economic phenomenon (see Kagan et al., 2022). These types of psychology are interested in activism and political engagement in a way that barely gets acknowledged within mainstream psychology. They reject, in general, the established quantitative processes that resonate with medical and scientific models that dominate theories and methods within mainstream psychology and therefore dominate practices and educational programmes at universities. Critical and community psychology on paper would appeal to disabled people and other marginalised groups because they are psychologies that have a vision of empowerment and inclusion. However, whilst critical/community psychology and other relatable psychologies provide routes away from an oppressive type of psychology, critical/community psychology does not hold the same influences that traditional disciplines within mainstream psychology have such as clinical, forensic, and neuropsychology's, signifying that despite the hope, critical/community psychology might bring, psychology overall will then continue to be viewed as an oppressive psychology. This then raises questions about what psychology could mean or not, with the label of 'psychology' or not.

Whilst I suggest that the definitions and meanings of psychology need to be redefined and refashioned, to become a psychology that connects with disabled people and other groups, that does not mean that what might encompass the 'psychological' or 'psychology' should be ignored or entirely rejected. I have referred to Watermeyer (2012) earlier in the book who made some useful points relating to this by pointing out that to address ideologies and power that are inherently disablist. Therefore, any kind of emancipation needs to happen by understanding power at all levels to understand the intersubjective norms, beliefs, and values that operate, to ensure justice does not prevail and exclusionary practices remain. So, whilst from a disability studies perspective, this would suggest that psychology is pathologising and medicalising, to arguably understand this and change this, we must 'go inside' and understand more about why it is disabling to unpack the subjective and intersubjective spaces that subordination can be understood (also see Watermeyer & Swartz, 2008). By doing so, psychology can then draw on other disciplines and perspectives to make sense of the subjectivities taking place that are disabling such as feminism and liberatory models associated with community psychologies at different levels. Also, the ideas of Freire (1970) and Martin-Baro (1994) can be used in relating to developing critical dialogues and becoming aware of oppression and the tools that make oppression happen which disabled people face in their homes, day centres, hospitals, and prisons as well as in less obvious places where disablism happens in shops, in parks, workplaces, and in relationships. This may help to get to the heart of the oppression and understand it more and begin to challenge it. Watermeyer (2012) suggests that we should avoid using 'broad brush strokes' at dismissing disciplines like psychology as oppressive without critical engagement; then, the easy rejections of such disciplines as medicalising are not seeing the possibilities of change and the opportunities that might bring to making changes for the better. Instead, cooperation across professionals and disciplines can ensure that everyone can make a valuable contribution to a re-understanding and changeable discipline. To go 'inside' the experiences of the lives of disabled people also means that psychology as we know it cannot continue. By empathising and understanding the lives of disabled people, it would mean that psychology in all its simplicities, reductionism, and logicism would have to become something different because those intersubjective experiences would turn psychology upside down. A critical posthumanities perspective would emphasise the pluralities and vitalism that make up the experiences of disabled people and this contrasts with the psychology that we have become to 'know' for a long time.

In that respect, we should see the opportunities for disabled people to be able to enact change in the community using the resources psychology can bring and prioritise the stories of disabled people in communities so that identities can emerge and be central to a psychology that is prepared to act and make a difference. This could lead to stronger relational dynamics of personal and institutional experiences of disabled people and the roles cultural meanings have on forging identities, and how these identities can be respected and add value to psychological knowledge, a move away from psychologising and pathologising. In addition, the disablist world can be challenged with the knowledge and insights from psychologists in collaboration with disabled people, going beyond the entrenched individual level of analysis that is a central tenet of mainstream psychology, which might go some way to challenging normalisation and its effects on stereotyping, labelling, and self-fulfilling prophecies. Consequently, psychology as we know it has a lot to offer, whether that is mainstream psychology or mainstream/critical community psychology, but the potential here also means that psychology would not be as we know it and cannot be as we know it for this to happen because the powerful experiences, expertise, and skills of disabled people would change psychology.

That being said, I question the meaning, definition, and the word of 'psychology' and ironically, I do not stop talking about it, and this would suggest that the idea of dismissing it all together is not possible. However, by stretching, playing around with, and grabbing psychology like rainbow coloured playdough and hitting it around, psychology could be refashioned or taken away as it is to become something that is fit for purpose for disabled people. Where psychology can gain so much from the qualities, skills, and experiences psychologists have to offer, but in genuine collaboration with them, redefining and relabelling a becoming psychology. Disabled people should be at the heart of this playing around with psychology rather than being its outcome of success if someone has been diagnosed with a problem, to then end up in a cycle of permanent control by 'person-centred' systems that are inherently disablist and old-fashioned. Our mis-/understandings of disabled people like our definitions of 'human' have been closed-off and self-contained, ensuring that there continues to be a binary between disabled and non-disabled and human and non/sub-human. A critical posthumanities view could ensure that the ambiguities, multiplicities, and complexities of what makes us who we are, are not ignored. A decentring of this and thinking about disabled people and humans all round as assemblages rather than fixations can begin to shift our thinking about what the study of psychology can become, and maybe psychology can really become dynamic, intersect, and reconfigure itself in a way that is influenced by experts of 'humanhood' such as disabled people. Those famous words that resonate with so many disability studies scholars of 'nothing about us without us' is still important today (see Charlton, 1998), but the 'us' must be everything and about everyone.

The ontology of becoming means that we are forever in flux, and we can see that in the labels, pathologising, technologising, medicalising, and psychologising of disabled people through the decades, but that means it is often changing in a negative way, and psychology has played its part in that (Goodley & Lawthom 2005a). For instance, the labels that are applied to disabled people have changed (handicap, spastic, mental retardation), yet the meaning behind these labels and the effects of these labels are as negative as they have ever been. If our understanding of what 'human' is and what the 'psych' or study of behaviour and mind was to change, then how we view disabled people might just change for the better too. And this is the problem with psychology, psychology changes at the surface level, but never appears to really change in a way that is transformative, and yet people and the world is forever in flux, which implies that psychology as we know it cannot exist and is not fit for purpose in representing the intersubjectivities and diverse identities that disabled people and other marginalised groups experience. As I suggested earlier in the book, psychology needs to redefine and reposition itself into a new-materialistic position because by doing so, it can be more effective, creative, and adaptable towards the urges, needs, identities, and positionalities of disabled people in our world. A new kind of 'posthuman community psychology' can emerge that is open minded and flexible about ever-changing contexts and meanings of humanhood, and this would be more beneficial to the lives of disabled people than what we understand psychology to currently be. A becoming companion species is not about us all becoming one blob of cells, squashed together as one life form that becomes meaningless and reduces the celebration of difference, diversity, and originality. Instead, a becoming psychology can be one and different at the same time, because that is how it is anyway, if you take away the barriers that prioritise class, money, economics, survival of the fittest, that have had negative impacts on both disabled people, other marginalised people, and in fact, everyone, in some way or another (see Chapter 1 for more analysis around 'becoming').

The word and meanings behind 'psychology' is a barrier for disabled people, and the traditional roots and development of mainstream psychology and critical/community psychologies in part ensure that psychology does not permeate into the lives of disabled people in a way that is empowering and inclusive. But to make this happen, psychology can emerge in new ways that might help to make disabled people smile when they hear the word or be a go to place where disabled people feel empowered and that they can share their expertise in collaboration with professionals in a way that is not tokenistic and intimidating. Psychology as we know it does not bring smiles to the faces of disabled people and itself is a barrier to change, therefore a rethinking of what 'psychology' can become would be refreshing and revolutionary for disabled people.

A becoming companion species – Disabilities are everything or no more?

In Chapter 5, I posited that for psychology to change or be redefined in its current form, we must think about how our communities work. For disabled people, they know how communities work because they are essentially disablist from top to bottom, and in many ways, sexist, racist, and ageist, and this means that for a disabled person who has multiple identities, like we all have, they will face further marginalisation and exclusionary practices and so maybe they are the real experts in critical/community psychology and psychology all round. The idea of a posthuman community psychology could not emerge unless disabilities are considered a way of life that affects everyone and this is understood by acknowledging and confronting the powerful disablist structures that are enshrined on societies through financialisaton, elite classes, and mostly dominate white, heterosexual, male, and wealthy identities.

The main approaches in psychology have set out how humans should think, feel, and behave, or this is how humans think, feel, and behave, within rigid structures of thinking in parallel with dominant neoliberal and western systems of finance, a way of thinking and life that is not competent with how disabled people think, feel, and behave. Society and psychology as we know it is rooted in disablist entrenchments that ensure that they are viewed and treated as sub-human, different in a way that it is not positive, and for a becoming posthuman community psychology to emerge, a recognition of companionships, relatedness, and accompaniment might go some way in reducing the inherent disablist ways of life that are sometimes clear and obvious and brutal and in other ways, subtle, intersubjective, and unseen. Therefore, the idea of a 'becoming companion of species' involves a move to a co-evolution (see Nayar, 2014) where there is recognition and action taken that considers that we share our communities, world, and beyond with ecosystems to life processes of all kinds alongside our developments of technology, which help to make us who we are and what we become, whatever that might be. Indeed, this is already happening because during these times of genetic engineering, technological advancements, and biomedical developments, disabled people have been at the heart of that for good and bad reasons, ensuring that their expertise and insights are at a level that psychologists cannot reach in the same way, for example, the use of technology for people who are deaf, for soldiers who have been amputated and received new technologically infused limbs, or the specialist technology in special education needs schools for autistic people. Technology and disabilities come together, understanding biomedical and genetic engineering comes hand-in-hand with understanding disabilities too, but that is often forgotten because of the sub-human category disabled people are placed within. A becoming companion of species would not be about transcending experts over novices, normal over abnormal, or strong over weak, but a companionship that co-evolves is a sensible way to view the changing nature of disabilities and humanhood. Mainstream psychology in its current form is behind that advancement and remains smoke screened by its arrogance that it has moved with the times, but this is not the experiences of disabled people, who are always a step ahead.

For disabled people, the idea of co-evolvement in our communities would be refreshing. The distinctions between the complex binaries that they face when they are judged ensure that there is a lack of awareness, interconnections, and mutual understandings between people, and this can only strengthen the linear, out of date theoretical positions of mainstream psychology that is dominated by biomedical and logical empiricist thinking.

Nayar's 'companion species' that is becoming and something that becomes a way of life to form a multispecies citizenship implies that the scientific and psychologising of disabilities as we know it would not exist. This would not mean that there would be a rejection of a critical realist perspective that people do need help and support. Disabled people need care and support that might be different to some other people, but instead disabled people would just be people rather than a segregated and indifferent group that gets petted down one minute as tragic victims and then the next minute is on the end of violent attacks and being spat at by bullies. We must think about humanhood in different ways and that can be done through being open-minded and being interconnected with disabled people, who are arguably already posthumans and can provide better insights into how a posthuman community psychology could work (see Goodley, Lawthom & Runswick-Cole, 2014).

Similar to Nayar (2014), I have posited that a becoming companion species fits well with a becoming posthuman community psychology because from that, a 'posthuman citizenship' may emerge that encapsulates the ever-changing nature of life. Disabled people are positioned to understand this better because there is always acknowledgement that their bodies and brains are changing, depicted as something often abnormal in our communities, when in fact, all our bodies and brains are always changing. Therefore, a posthuman citizenship can help us understand disabled people not as a separate entity that is used in science for outcomes, but one that is embodied and interconnects with the environment, and that we can only understand people, living things, and our communities or one whole community through the intersectional connections that can only be understood in context with how we interact with our world, technologies, and biology. In other words, a companion species for disabled people and all people would be one that is becoming where all people care for one another for mutually beneficial reasons that go beyond the binaries that are applied to disabled people and their identities, to something that is less discriminatory and exclusionary, and where accompaniment is the way of life for real survival and happiness.

Changing the dynamic of psychology and the world around it or within it for disabled people would not be easy. As I have previously said, psychology and psychologists are not easily going to give up billions of pounds of research money or relinquish their positions of power to develop into a 'psychology' that is mutual, interconnected, and less alienating for disabled people. However, it would be mutually beneficial for them and for disabled people for psychology to be a space that is dynamic, diverse, liberating, and shrouded in humility (see Kagan et al., 2021). A becoming companion of species can revitalise the ways, approaches, and methods that have been used across the spectrum of psychologies to something that is genuinely empowering and inclusive for all disabled people, and this is a choice psychologists could make, if they wanted to. What would this mean for disabled people? In psychology's current format and structure, disabled people can only continue to be a 'subject' in an experiment, be used in a tokenistic way or be convinced that participation in a research project where they can do some drawing 'will do them good', whereas a posthuman community psychology would and should seek to turn that upside down. Psychology could change to something that is fit for purpose for disabled people through their expertise, insights, skills, and enthusiasms which can connect with established psychologists. Yes, we are all face disabling or exclusionary circumstances at some point, and the cynic might say in that case psychologists are and will be disabled anyway, so keep it as it is, but that is with a positionality of education, wealth, power, and position in a way that most disabled people never experience. This means that a becoming companion species must be more than just about being a 'psychologist' or a 'participant'. A posthuman community psychology, with a similar outlook as some critical disability thinkers, means that a becoming companion of species is something that is inclusive, feminist, queer, scientific, technological, earth, and cosmos (see Goodley & Runswick-Cole, 2016; Goodley et al., 2017). I would say that this encapsulates the new people we keep becoming and the relationship between what psychology can become and disabled people need that changing outlook that goes beyond the stale format of contemporary psychology but whilst making use of what all psychologies have to offer.

Assemblage approach to care and community – Beyond 'person'-centred 'care'

To explore how we understand psychology, our communities, how they function, and what they contribute towards people's lives, especially the most marginalised such as disabled people, there must be a conversation about rethinking 'person' 'centred' 'care'. My own experiences of working with disabled people in care home environments and alongside their care workers, managers, and working with charities in the community have led me to reflect on what a disaster it is for many disabled people, with some ameliorative and tokenistic positive changes, genuine care, and facilitation that leads to empowerment here and there. The environments of care homes, day centres, small businesses that promote empowerment and change and other places such as museums and medical centres, and other places are inherently disabling and promote subtle and obvious forms of disablism. To what extent do disabled people have choices? Where is their expertise in all this? Where are their skills being applied? This is very difficult to see happening in a way that is wholly inclusive and participative because these systems are top-down, profit-driven (same approach even when not-for-profit), and white-driven ensuring that the whole set-up of the care system, and I speak from a UK context, is not fit for purpose for disabled people. Of course, I have worked in these communities with my own agenda such as wanting to complete research, to take something from disabled people, albeit with maybe the naïve intentions of changing their world for the better. But this arrogance and position of power do not reflect the changing nature of humanhood that I have explored in this book, nor does it invoke feelings of care, empowerment, and inclusivity.

For disabled people, there are few alternatives, and many are chained down, psychologically, and physically, to a system that is caring in words, but not in actions. Critical realists would say that care homes and day centres are needed because for many these places have been places of safety and empowerment and people can get the round the clock care that they need. I am not saying that this is wrong, but there are consistent cases of abuse, disempowerment, and exclusionary practices that ensure that for many disabled people, the 'care experience' is not caring at all, and ameliorative initiatives and worded mentions in policy is not going to make a difference or change the disablist systems that encapsulate the care system. However, the idea of an assemblage system of care might go some way to develop a becoming companion species where disabled people can be genuine powerbrokers and leaders in the care system where their voices lead to action and that the focus is on voice and being, rather than being objectified as sub-human and not functional in line with neoliberalist ideologies. An assemblage approach to care and community would mean mutual collaboration and care that decides what makes people happier, respected, and loved. If this was to happen, the 'person-centredness' to care as we have come to know it and has been around for decades, could not be applied anymore and is not in line with the changing ways of being for humans. Person-centred approaches in different respects are out of date for disabled people because they are inconsistent with how people are becoming. A becoming posthuman community psychology approach would think about care as assemblages where difference, the complexities, and intersubjectivities of care and support for community members need to be transformed and not tied into neoliberal and capitalist ideologies of costs, outcomes, and 'evidence-based' initiatives that are top-down and disempowering.

The biomedical nature of person-centred care ensures that the strong values that were proposed by the People First Movement such as their basic rights, need for accessibility, making their own decisions, being empowered, and having choices (see Griffiths, 2022) are not in line and seem worlds apart from one another. Person-centred care is still primarily about cure and treatment and aims to keep people balanced and occupied, ensuring disabled voices are non-existent, unless a funding bid needs to be rubber stamped with 'disabled voices' to make it look better. The Rogerian approach and other humanist approaches in nature provide powerful ideas around congruent relationships that are meant to be at the heart of person-centred approaches, but this does not exist for most disabled people, rendering person-centred care essentially a structure and way of life that suits the same people who dominate political power. A posthuman community psychology resonates with the ideas from Braidotti (2013) and other critical posthumanity writers that the body is intersectional and made up of many codes, not just biological and sociological. For example, care systems are underpinned by biomedical outlooks that see the body as purely 'biological', when in fact how we use our bodies, judge them, play with them, care for them, are influenced to how we are connected to what is in context, ensuring the body is political, and not just cells and bones. The 'body' in the care system is something to 'sort out', that feeling of as long as someone's bum is wiped and you can stick a plate of food under their chin, then 'job done'. But this transaction or exchange of care (see Toro & Martiny, 2020) demonstrates the fears, exaggerations and curiosities of a body that is enshrined in complex ethics, values, and politics, and for a 'disabled' judged body, whether of disgust, fantasy or excitement, it ensures that the simplistic approach to person-centred care ignores that complicated exchange of glances, staring, touch, emotional connections, intrigue, and fear. Ultimately, the body that is considered disabled is considered to be something that someone would want to change, needs to change, needs to be smoothed over, but that is static, permanent, and immoveable, when in fact the body is dynamic (Shildrick, 2007, 2009). The person-centred approach to care is about normative bodies and brains that need a bit of care rather than seeing people in context of their multiple identities and their expertise, skills, and awareness of the world. The post-conventionalism of Shildrick's work further highlights that the body is a cultural and corporeal production and so a disabled person' body can challenge how we view normative bodies, but that in turn from a critical posthumanities perspective means that bodies are much more than biology. They are interconnected and intersect with everything else, and the person-centredness of care ideology is poor at considering people and their beings in this way.

An assemblage approach to care and community for disabled people might mean a deeper understanding of the many factors that contextualise care for disabled people. The changes, differences, becomings at the heart of how we care and how we think we should care should not be made linear and boxed off and, instead, should be considered in all its ambiguities and not set within humanised boundaries. Tokenistic decisions relating to including disabled people in their care are ameliorative at best. The critics might say that this is better than in the past when this was not taking place, but it is hardly taking place now and has not led to the transformation of the care needed to meet complex lives disabled people face. Disabled people need to be within and alongside everyone where we will all need care, at the heart of decision-making that is not set in stone but is fluid and ongoing to stimulate real empowerment. There is a need for a move away from the ongoing medical model of disability that continues to have the overarching gaze on how we understand disabilities and disabled people, and humanhood and what we can become.

Relational methods, approaches, and tools – Whatever makes you happy

The real joy I got when I have worked in the community or when working with colleagues and students over the years has always been when there is a creative edge to the work or actions or participation that takes place. How can I not be excited about witnessing and hearing the poetic words of gay disabled people who want to express their love and invoke humour or when students tell me about how they facilitate art and crafts with autistic children. How can I not enjoy the excitement of a disabled adult going to the cinema to watch a Marvel film to then go home and imagine themselves as their hero or invent their own hero or when someone shows me their photographs on their phone about their experiences of being with nature or how they have created and organised their garden. How can I not feel engaged and intrigued about these creations and stories when they feel like moments of hope for those individuals and participants that despite the difficulties and challenges they face, they find their own methods and tools and use them to tell their stories, to act and promote their feelings of how they understand the world around them.

This is a far cry away from the experiments, interviews, questionnaires, and observational type studies that make up most of the research, practices, and approaches of psychologists. Yes, there are more and more tools, digital and non-digital that are being used, more ways to use arts and craft and more visual methods to use, but the premise in most psychological research relates to the same methods that invoke input and output approaches that psychologises the data, personalities, actions, and words of their participants. Again, I acknowledge that I have been no different and many critical/community psychologists have been no different, but I am not saying this is completely wrong and needs to change. Those traditional methods, quantitative or qualitative in nature or both, have played a part in helping promote the voices of disabled people from time to time and they have helped to provide some structure and decision-making that helps disabled people. However, psychological methods, approaches, and tools have ensured that the voices of disabled people, their experiences, stories, humour, and ambitions have been stifled away from the scientific premises of easy and concise conclusions, that fit in with the expectations of funders and with the expectations that have been at the heart of modern and contemporary psychology for 150 years. If a posthuman community psychology was a way of becoming for disabled people, then the tools that are available and will become available have to be accessible and open-to-all. Having a voice makes people happy and the tools at the disposal of psychologists and other professionals can help to bring happiness, cooperation and produce rich, creative, inspiring data that can get to the very heart of the experiences of disabled people. It is an opportunity to promote voices in a way never seen in psychology. Is it time for psychologists to turn to disabled people and ask them for help on how to use tools, methods, and approaches that will take psychology to a different space of becoming?

A posthuman community psychology where we are co-evolving with relational methods, approaches, and tools that promote voice may help us to express and become identities that humans might not have been before. This suggests that we are very much in a posthuman period, but psychology, despite having the technology, methods, and influences at its disposal, is still stuck in old-fashioned ways that are not as becoming for disabled people. Condie and Richards (2022) have already discussed the idea of a 'digital community psychology', which is focused on critical/community psychology's poor record in promoting the digital with marginalised groups, as opposed to mainstream psychology's prominent use of digital technology albeit arguably in a way that seeks to manipulate and control. Yet, there is much potential for disabled people here because just holding a phone or laptop and pressing buttons can be empowering, but to discover ways on how to use it to promote your voice, creativity, and take action, could be a way that brings disabled people to the forefront of research and activism. Yes, people will say what about people who cannot read or write or cannot afford this technology, but the world is increasingly becoming technologised and we are all connected to this in some way, and there is no way of getting away from it. A posthuman and new-materialist perspective on how we understand and use technology can bridge the gap between societal levels and local community levels and how we understand disabilities, making it relational and interconnected, where change can take place when needed to challenge social justice issues.

A posthuman community psychology that intersects and is open to all perspectives about how we might think about humans and psychology and communities needs to be able to explore and interrogate and engage with tools and ideas that can lead to us becoming. Imagine what insights, expertise, and skills that we can all learn from if relational methods of research and practice are handled by disabled people. This is likely to be inclusive and empowering in a way that you could never experience in an interview room that might remind people of when they were assessed and ignored, or a questionnaire that ensures an opinion cannot be given or an experiment where you are number 2 rather than Jenny.

Deideologising disablist ideas and decolonising the psychologised gaze on disabled people

For a posthuman community psychology to emerge, there must be an acceptance that what we understand to be psychology needs to be decolonised and deideologised, and this makes sense if the proposal is that mainstream and critical/community psychology in its current form is not suitable, and maybe never was, especially for disabled people. Similar to different writers in psychology, mainstream, or critical/community, critical disability studies scholars have written about the stifling nature of colonialism and its effects on disabled people, and they would seek a process of decolonisation to extinguish the dominance of the psychologised gaze on disabled people (Grech, 2015; Watermeyer, 2019). I have spoken about how a becoming companion species would not be able to emerge as a form of co-evolvement and mutuality if psychology and many other institutions remained colonial and driven by traditional ideologies of how we view people and the world. A decolonised psychology means the psychology as we think we know it does not exist and would reduce the inherent whiteness of psychology that permeates through disability studies.

Fanon's work (1952, 1967) on highlighting the politics in psychology is still relevant today and relevant for disabled people because 'disability' is political and embroiled in power, in obvious and subtle ways. Fanon's work epitomises the need to explore the intersubjective experiences of everyday life for people such as those with disabilities and by doing so, there is more chance for a progressive politics that encompass values of relationality, interconnectedness, and accompaniment. The need to reclaim, refashion, and centre the concerns of disabled people who have directly affected by colonialism is important to understand the experiences of those people but provides added insights into those people who are also disabled and have multiple identities that are promoted in a negative way, a way that is not mutual or beneficial for anyone. A posthuman community psychology that encompasses the open-mined and fluid ideas within critical posthumanities would reject the dominance of whiteness and neoliberalism and become a transformative state of becoming that avoids the binaries that have established humanhood for a long time in our thinking about what being 'human' means.

To decolonise means to deideologise, and Freire's (1970) principles relating to conscientisation are useful because we become aware, understand the nature of power and the complexities of being disabled and the identities that intersect with that identity and how it fits into the world better. The more 'disabled' you become the more aware of exclusionary practices you are, and this awareness can be helped through the methods, tools, and approaches I have previously discussed, such as through digital technology, the awareness will bring more hope and resilience to challenge systems and change those systems. Yes, that 'awareness' has been there for a long time and can be seen in the civil rights movements over the past 60 years, but it is difficult to have awareness and to know how to change things and have a genuine voice when encased in structures that do the opposite such as care systems, medical institutions, and workplaces. Through conscientisation, disabled people would feel the empowering effects of awareness and dialogue as the potential to challenge established institutes and powerbases like psychology, and by challenging psychology, there is hope it can be fit for purpose or reimagined as something that is becoming and liberating. Similar to the becoming critical disability studies in recent years, posthuman community psychology can be a transdisciplinary space, which reaches out to different perspectives, helping psychology to be a space that becomes open-minded and is prepared to intersect more with other philosophical perspectives including postmodernist (Shakespeare & Corker, 2002), post-structuralist (Tremain, 2005), and posthuman (Braidotti, 2013; Goodley et al., 2014) thinking, and by doing so, starts to reinvent itself as a becoming psychology that will let go of the shackles of colonialism and all that posits colonialism. This may help psychology to move beyond the material dominance of scientific psychology that remain static, in a way that the social model of disability had become

(Meekosha & Shuttleworth, 2009) and think in ways that are queer, discursive, cultural, and relational (see Tremain, 2005; Shildrick, 2007, 2009; Roets & Goodley, 2008; Campbell, 2008; Slater, 2015). Meekosha and Shuttleworth (2009) suggested that critical disability studies are important because they build on the multiple interdisciplinarities that encompass disability studies, whilst continuing to incorporate relevant aspects of the social model of disability as well as listening to work emerging from the global South (see Grech and Goodley, 2012), but psychology could do with going through the same experiences and it might go some way to decolonise and deideologise itself.

'Critical' disability studies then concern going beyond the established ways of thinking about disabilities, not always just to reject what has been said before, but indeed to inform and build on what has been said before, so that our understanding of disabilities is ever-changing and ever-evolving through multiple processes and nuances, intersecting across multiple identities relating to class, genders, sexualities, and race. The epistemological and ontological developments of disability studies, informed by activism, voices of the disabled as well as the professionals and organisations, good or bad, are continuing to make contributions to allow the gaze of a critical disability studies thinker to be more open-minded and see humanity and disability in a deeper way than before. This is parallel with the ideas that have emerged from critical posthumanities, and if psychology was also to be a posthuman psychology and be like this, then it enhances the possibilities, experiences, the empowerment, and identities of disabled people and can contribute to making psychology a force for good that is in line with the becoming nature of being in the world.

Beyond and within the 'psych' – Working together means understanding the effects of disabilities better

I have posited through this book that psychology has many identities and in that sense is an example of posthumanism in action. Psychology in certain respects has encompassed different psychologies, brought in different methods and technologies, and become a powerful beast in terms of the expertise, money, and power it has over institutions and ways of life. In a way, that was not the case when modern psychology emerged in the later part of the 19th century. Yet, it somehow has remained the same, the roots of psychology still uphold the psychology we now know in the 21st century. Why is this a problem? By remaining at the general individual level of analysis, focusing on the 'psych', it means that how we view beings and their contexts and what they can become remains static and narrow. In this instance, it should then be no surprise that the experiences of disabled people when matched up with psychologists or psychology in some way are wholly negative because as I have discussed we cannot see humans in a simplistic way, nor can disabled people be viewed in this way.

A posthuman community psychology would graze between different disciplines, philosophies, and professions, in a way that the field of disability studies has done for years. With psychology deeply rooted in science, logic and reason and only with touches of cross wiring with disciplines such as sociology, cultural studies and many more, then it just reinforces itself and its power on how we should view humans and how we should view disabled people and that needs to change. A posthuman community psychology would give itself away to forward thinking new ideas and creations that emerge as humans emerge, as disabled people emerge, and this would be a psychology that people could engage with and love and see as something that is about them and not about the same kind of people doing the same kind of things in psychology that have been done for a long time. This new-materialist way of being means disabled people, with psychologists and other professionals and disciplines, can be who they are and want to be and others, a lived experience, felt within, and an embodiment that connects with technology, society, and discursion, an assemblage of all kinds of things and beings (see Fox & Alldred, 2017). To be within and around an ever-changing assemblage means that the 'psych' and the 'ology' in its simplicity are not real or connected to us, but assemblages that intersect and interconnect with other ideas, disciplines, and ways of being and thinking enhance how we might go back and view the 'psych'. This links back to the ideas of Deleuze and Guattari (1987) where in the process of becoming we are plural, uneven, and messy and that the changing nature of the mind and body are related to emerging and changing assemblages that will keep becoming.

If we see disabilities and psychologies in the context of becoming, then the complexities of becoming mean stepping within and out of psychology, so a psychology that is not pegged within reductionist boundaries. Psychology is already in many ways demonstrating its worth when connecting with disciplines and crossing over into new ideas, which is a positive way to understand the complicated lives that disabled people face. Yet, as I have said in this book, it remains the same somehow, ensuring that disabled people will continue to experience and feel the potential that psychology can offer beyond the lab and interview rooms where old-fashioned styles of psychologising and diagnosing of labels takes place rather than actually experiencing the potential into action. If disabled people are entangled within assemblages influenced by many factors that are ever-changing, then to psychologise through basic research methods and Likert scales is counterproductive and can only enhance the disablist structures that disabled people face within psychology and its associate disciplines, underpinned by medical models of disability. A posthuman community psychology would go beyond the hardened boundaries of idealised modernity to a decentred, fluid, and interconnected phenomenon.

Justice for all – Marginalising disabilities is an injustice for all

A posthuman community psychology, where a becoming companion of species emerges, needs justice to be at the centre, where the voices of disabled people are centred along with other marginalised voices, which all round, psychology across the spectrum of psychologies has been a disaster. For justice for all to prevail, a space needs to open up that is becoming where disabled people feel wanted and cared for in a way that that connects with them and all other beings. But, for social justice to prevail, psychology needs to give up its partial humanist stance on 'inclusion' (for some, psychology has never been humanistic) and be more in tune with the uneven and flexible critical posthumanist stance that has guided the development of the ideas behind a posthuman community psychology. With inclusion comes social justice, and disabled people have maybe only ever known this in bits and pieces like other marginalised groups, people, and other beings. We can reflect on the new-materialist idea that the humanist 'self' is based on separation of mind from matter (see Barad, 2007), and how this links in with epistemological positionings of positivism, structuralism, and logical empiricism, all of which underpin modern and contemporary psychology, but by doing so, ensures that inclusion and therefore social justice, which affects us all is left in the trash outside those scientific boundaries. The rationalised 'self' that under-scores what humanism, humanistic psychology, critical, and community psy-chologies represent raises questions not just about what humans and beings are in an always changing world of technology, cultures, identities, and biol-ogies, but this raises questions about life itself and what it means to be dis-abled. In this respect, a posthuman community psychology would embrace a social justice for all because it would be a move towards a new-materialist viewpoint that is affirmative and situated (Ulmer, 2017) in a way that looks at alternative ways of understanding inclusion and social justice. This is nec-essary when considering some basic facts in the UK in 2021 relating to the experiences of disabled people, which provides a surface-level overview of the day-to-day social misjustices that take place compared to 'non-disabled' people (Office of National Statistics, 2021). For example:

- Disabled people less likely to have a degree compared to others.
- Disabled people less likely to be employed.
- Disabled people less likely to own their own home.
- Disabled people's well-being is lower and are more likely to feel lonelier, exasperating their mental health. With life satisfaction being poorer.
- Disabled people less likely to participate in civic engagement and be con-sulted about changes that directly affects them in the community.
- Disabled people more likely to face hate crime, anti-social behaviour, nuisance behaviour and neighbours.

This list could be increased further when thinking about subtle and blatant ableist educational, financial, religious, political, and business orientated systems that expunge difference across global societies. Other marginalised groups and people have experienced similar, and aspects of this will be experi-enced by 'non-disabled' people and beings too. However, the above statements ensure that disabled people face social injustice not periodically, or now and again, but it remains a permanent state of being. This is despite what a critical posthumanities outlook might suggest that disabilities are always changing and moving, ensuring that there is a double whammy of disablist ways of being within our societies, whilst bodies, minds, beings are always on the move. In addition, the statistics above do not highlight the double, triple and more discriminations that disabled people face with their multiple identities as women, gay, trans, older, younger, and other identities, or the one billion people plus around the world who identify as being disabled who face extreme poverty, damaging effects of climate change, unhealthy, and dangerous living conditions, for many no medical care, education, and total social exclusion. Why has psychology not made in-roads into changing these circumstances? A critical realist psychologist might posit that this is not what psychology is about and psychology is not placed to make differences on this scale, and yet, psychology has all the power, money, influences, and skills to make in-roads in changing the world for the better. A posthuman community psychology must seek to change the world and not just take from what is already within our communities there and leave that loose data behind when finished. For disabled people to have permanent social justice and inclusion, then everyone must play a part and psychology is placed at micro and macro levels within communities and societies to contribute to making positive changes that are powerful and transformative. A psychology that embraces a new-materialist idea of going beyond the rigidity of biological systems, to one that affects us all, will have profound effects on disabled people, such as biotechnological developments, advances in genetics or climate change, and psychology can become and already is within an entanglement of a 'onto-epistemology' where entities co-exist and co-evolve relationally (Barad, 2008). Psychology becoming an assemblage that is material-discursive of all things always in flux might go some way into being affective in contributing to social justice that brings happiness for disabled people, and therefore, for all beings.

Summary

This final chapter reviewed and mirrored the ideas of a 'posthuman community psychology' in the context of how it might look for disabled people, whether it is about changing the structures and institutions in society or whether it concerns the daily practices and behaviours of how disabled people experience life. The narrative has been formed to be as positive as possible, but I am conscious again that this is one set of reflections, guided by different experiences and insights from the literature and practice, and a disabled writer with many identities and experiences might have a different view. However, I set out that for disabled people, all round, psychology, and psychologists have been met with suspicions, hate, and mistrust. That does not mean that for everyone, the experiences have been poor, but there is a disconnect with the ever-changing nature of what 'disability' means, whereas at the same time, psychology is mostly stuck in how it approaches, works, and engages with disabled people in the same way as psychologists would have done a hundred years ago. There needs to be a psychology that is compassionate and moves with the times as disabled people have moved with the times, and maybe the ideas that I have reflected upon for a post-human community psychology could add to those debates and conversations. That being said, psychology is not going to relinquish its power, nor are the neoliberal and capitalist structures within psychology and society going to change any time soon, to help a society become one that is relational and interconnected in a way that ensures justice for all. But that should not stop new ideas, creations, imaginations, and activism emerging to promote a becoming companion species where multiple identities will only keep emerging and wanting new ways to become, where disabled people can teach psychology and psychologists much about what that means.

Overall summary of the book

The book has explored some big topics and only flicked the edges of each big topic, but enough to paint a sketch of where modern psychology came from (my interpretation), where contemporary psychology arguably is now and what it could become, at least from my perspective. I began the book with a futuristic and technological outlook of how someone might be diagnosed with ASD in the future, alluding to the fact that the clinical, objective, and labelling voice of the 'judge' was not just one for the future, but that pathologising and psychologising voice has been present for a long time for disabled people and other marginalised groups and likely to continue. This would suggest that we are not a becoming set of beings, and that futuristic outlook is not where we need to go if psychology embraces change either. The book is not seeking to provide an answer or a set of commandments of how life should be and what it will become. The book is a series of reflections that is opening debates that seek to go beyond the set boundaries that psychology, of all kinds, has established and to try to think boldly about how we can cross those barriers in a way that is co-evolving with all psychologies and beyond, and acknowledges that psychology needs to change as communities and people change.

   The book began by setting out some of the core ideas that underpin an ever-changing set of ideas that have emerged from critical posthumanities particularly influenced by Braidotti and Nayar. The guiding ideas that emerged helped me to think about psychology and what it could become and why on the one hand psychology has been in a state of becoming and yet somehow remains the same. I considered not just mainstream psychology in this exploration but also considered the 'humanist' psychologies such as mainstream and critical community psychology, which provide a critical analysis of psychology, communities, societies, and the world, but have made limited in-roads into changing psychology, whilst mainstream psychology continues to become popular, stronger, and influential. Nevertheless, although mainstream psychology is rooted in old-fashioned scientific principles of positivism, post-positivism, and empiricism, mainstream psychology like critical and community psychologies, have made contributions that have helped to save people's lives, helped to empower people, and include people and contributed to policy and legislation that has helped to enhance people's lives and voices. However, psychology in all its formats has not gone as far has it can to change the world, which it has the potential to do, but it remains doggedly the same. A critical posthumanities influenced posthuman community psychology has provided some reflections on helping to think about how psychology can move forward. For example, through some vague ideas concerning:

1   Redefining or refashioning or removing psychology altogether.
2   A becoming companion species, where a cosmopolitan way of life goes beyond the Anthropocene.
3   An assemblage approach to care and community – if we are no longer the 'humans' we have always thought we were, then how can 'person-centred' care continue as it does?
4   The relational connections with methods, tools, and approaches to promote voices and activism.
5   The significance of decolonising and deideologising psychology to a psychology that is about mutual companionship.
6   Going beyond the 'psych' and embracing disciplines, approaches, ideas, philosophies in a way that psychology has never dared do before. Being imaginative and open to all things.
7   Justice for all because it cannot be just about ameliorative interventions helping one group or one person, one day or in one time, justice concerns all things and there is a role to play for all of us.

The extent to which these ideas are realistic and can be put into practice or to transform entrenched and complicated powerbases in our world and communities is very debatable. But in my queerying through this book, where my aim was not to be a prophet or a great philosophical thinker, I just reflected upon what could be, with hope and some imagination. As I suggested at the beginning of the book, some will say that too much is being considered in this book. I understand that, but I reiterate, as a psychologist, where the study of 'human' behaviour is at the heart of it, to be able to turn that upside down and think about it in the context of disabilities and other marginalised groups, and what it means to be human and to bring some hope that psychology can be a psychology for the people, whatever those people are, then trying to write about all that will be complicated. Similarly, would the voices of marginalised people have a different take on the narrative, I am sure they would. If I was not a privileged white man who lives a comfortable life compared to most would I have a different view, then I am sure that would be the case too, but I hope that by acknowledging this and queerying myself and positionalities that influence the narrative, it goes someway into making this narrative something that sounds as honest as it can be. The thought of a posthuman community psychology could be just another addition, or not, to the many critical perspectives on psychology, or more 'psychobabble' or a cheap version of 'critical community psychology', but it might just highlight at the minimal level no matter how convincing the ideas are or not, that psychology and critical/community psychology have entered a posthuman turn, or need to, as the world changes around those psychologies.

The book is dominated by a critical lens on mainstream psychology, and that should be no surprise from a critical community psychologist, but the ideas that emerge would suggest that all psychologies have a part to play in becoming a relational, diverse psychology for the people, working alongside dedicated and skilled professionals. To do that, psychology needs to be shaken and stirred, turned upside down, and start to go beyond tokenism and ameliorative action. It needs to be something that is a voice for people and real-life issues relating to social justice and climate change, working across disciplines, and applying digital, creative, and visual methods in a way that is empowering and inclusive beyond set research and clinical practice circles, and by doing so, it can decolonise and deideologise itself.

All psychologies have a part to play in becoming a psychology that is something for marginalised people to become happy about and rely on for care and support in a way that is relational, interconnected and plural. This is a move away from humanist ideals of 'self' and 'individualism' that stifle the becoming nature of being and this can be seen in other disciplines such as critical disability studies through a disability lens where much can be understood about how change can happen through the experiences of disabled people. People with disabilities in many respects still face the same stigma and marginalisation as they did hundreds of years ago, which is no exaggeration, and yet, they find themselves the pioneers of the technology that is available to help people with disabilities move, speak, hear, interpret in a way other humans have never been able to do. In this respect, we must seriously consider whether disabled people are in fact a glimpse into what a posthuman future might look like. We can learn from disabled people and develop a world that gets rid of the chains of distinguishing who is disabled or not, to a world where people are just people, forever experiencing multiple assemblages and becoming rather than being defined from medical, psychologised, and politicised positions of power.

Psychology does have the potential to change and make a difference that is powerful and profound, but we have genuinely got to want that for it to happen, otherwise psychology will remain the same. Psychology should not be about the grim reapers that make up critical and community psychology, angry, and critical of everything, nor should it be driven and popularised by the same people who run governments, big businesses, banks, education, and other institutions, all of whom tend to be made up of mostly white, men, middle class and above, wealthy and heterosexual. Psychology, and all kinds of psychology and psychologists, need to be about co-evolvement, a becoming psychology that has the power, creativity, imagination, and skills to bring genuine equality and inclusion to beings and their communities.

References

Abrahams, T. (2017). Braidotti, Spinoza and Disability Studies after the Human. *History of the Human Sciences, 30*(5), pp. 86–103.

Akhurst, J. & Msomi, N. (2022). Building Partnerships for Community-Based Service-Learning in Poverty-Stricken and Systematically Disadvantaged Communities. In Kagan, C., Akhurst, J., Alfaro, J., Lawthom, R., Richards, M. & Zambrano, A. (eds.) *The Routledge International Handbook of Community Psychology.* New York: Routledge.

Adams, T.E. & Holman-Jones, S. (2011). Telling Stories: Reflexivity, Queer Theory, and Autoethnography. *Cultural Studies – Critical Methodologies, 11*(2), pp. 108–116.

Ahmed, S. (2006). *Queer Phenomenology: Orientations, Objects, Others.* Durham, NC: Duke University Press.

Albee, G.W. (1996). The Psychological Origins of the White Male Patriarchy. *Journal of Primary Prevention, 17*, pp. 75–97.

American Psychiatric Association. (2013). *Diagnostic and Statistical Manual of Mental Disorders* (5th ed.). American Psychiatric Association.

Angelique, H. (2011). Embodying Critical Feminism in Community Psychology: Unraveling the Fabric of Gender and Class. *Journal of Community Psychology, 40*(1), pp. 77–92.

Anthony, B. (2021). Implications of Telehealth and Digital Care Solutions during COVID-19 Pandemic: A Qualitative Literature Review. *Informatics for Health and Social Care, 46*(1), pp. 68–83.

Arnold, J. & Foncubierta, J.M. (2021). The Humanistic Approach. In Gregersen, T. & Mercer, S. (eds.) *The Routledge Handbook of the Psychology of Language, Learning and Teaching.* New York: Routledge.

Badmington, N. (2004). Mapping Posthumanism. *Environment and Planning, 36*(8), pp. 1344–1351.

Banister, P., Burman, E., Parker, I., Taylor, M. & Tindall, C. (1994). *Qualitative Methods in Psychology: A Research Guide.* Buckingham: Open University Press.

Barad, K. (2007). *Meeting the Universe Halfway: Quantum Physics and the Entanglement of Matter and Meaning.* Durham, NC: Duke University Press.

Barad, K. (2008). *Living in a Posthumanist Material World – Lessons from Schrodinger's Cat.* In Smelik, A. & Lykke, N. (eds.) *Bits of Life – Feminism at the Intersections of Media, Bioscience and Technology.* Seattle: University of Washington Press.

Barnes, C. (1991). *Disabled People in Britain and Discrimination: A Case for Antidiscrimination Legislation.* London: Hurst and Co. Ltd.

Barthes, R. (1957/2009). *Mythologies*. London: Penguin Books.

Bender, M.P. (1976). *Community Psychology*. London: Methuen.

Bennet, C., Anderson, L, Cooper, S., Hassol, L., Klein, D. & Rosenblum, G. (1966). *Community Psychology: A Report of the Boston Conference on the Education of Psychologists for Community Mental Health*. Boston, MA: Boston University.

Berger, P.L. & Luckmann, T. (1966). *The Social Construction of Reality: A Treatise in the Sociology of Knowledge*. New York: Doubleday & Company.

Bertelli, M.C., Rossi, M., Scuticchio, D. & Bianco, A. (2015). Diagnosing Psychiatric Disorders in People with Intellectual Disabilities: Issues and Achievements. *Advances in Mental Health and Intellectual Disabilities, 9*(5), pp. 230–242.

Blumberg, H.H., Hare, P.A. & Costin, A. (2006). *Peace Psychology: A Comprehensive Introduction*. Cambridge: Cambridge University Press.

Bolter, J.D. (2016). Posthumanism. In Jensen, K.B., Craig, R.T., Pooley, J.D. & Rothenbuhler, E.W. (eds.), *The International Encyclopaedia of Communication Theory and Philosophy*. Hoboken, NJ: Wiley.

Bostrom, N. (2002). When Machines Outsmart Humans. *Futures, 35*(7), pp. 759–764.

Bostrom, N. (2003a). Are You Living in a Computer Simulation. *Philosophical Quarterly, 53*(211), pp. 243–255.

Bostrom, N. (2003b). Human Genetic Enhancements: A Transhumanist Perspective. *Journal of Value Inquiry, 37*(4), pp. 493–506.

Botha, M. (2021). Critical Realism, Community Psychology, and the Curious Case of Autism: A Philosophy and Practice of Science with Social Justice in Mind. *Journal of Community Psychology*, https://onlinelibrary.wiley.com/doi/10.1002/jcop.22764.

Braidotti, R. (2006). Posthuman, All Too Human Towards a New Process Ontology. *Theory, Culture and Society, 23*(7–8), pp. 197–208.

Braidotti, R. (2010). The Politics of "Life Itself" and New Ways of Dying. In Coole, D. & Frost, S. (eds.) *New Materialisms: Ontology, Agency, and Politics* (pp. 201–218). Durham, NC: Duke University Press.

Braidotti, R. (2013). *The Posthuman*. Cambridge: Polity.

Braidotti, R. (2017). Critical Posthuman Knowledges. *South Atlantic Quarterly, 116*(1), pp. 83–96.

Braidotti, R. (2019). A Theoretical Framework for the Critical Posthumanities. *Theory, Culture & Society, 36*(6), pp. 31–61.

Braidotti, R. (2022). Posthuman Neo-materialisms and Affirmation. In Daigle, C. & McDonald, T.H. *Deleuze and Guattari to Posthumanism – Philosophies of Immanence*. Bloomsbury.

Brennan, J. (2020). Trust as a Test for Unethical Persuasive Design. *Philosophy & Technology, 34*(4), pp. 1–17.

Brett, G.S. (1921/2013). *A History of Psychology: Medieval & Early Modern Period, Volume 2*. New York: Routledge.

Brinkmann, S. (2017). Humanism after Posthumanism: Or Qualitative Psychology after the 'Posts'. *Qualitative Research in Psychology, 14*(2), pp. 109–130.

British Psychological Society (2022). Member Networks. https://www.bps.org.uk/member-networks

Bronfenbrenner, U. (1977). Toward an Experimental Ecology of Human Development. *American Psychologist, 32*(7), pp. 513–531.

Bugental, J.F.T. (1964). The Third Force in Psychology. *Journal of Humanistic Psychology, 4*(1), pp. 19–26.

Burman, E. (2018). Towards a Posthuman Developmental Psychology of Child, Families and Communities. In Fleer, M. & van Oers, B. (eds.) *International Handbook of Early Childhood Education*. The Netherlands: Springer.

Burr, V. (2015). *Social Constructionism* (3rd ed.). New York: Routledge.

Burton, M., Boyle, S., Harris, C. & Kagan, C. (2007). *International Community Psychology: History and Theories*. The Netherlands: Springer.

Butler, J. (1993). *Bodies that Matter: On the Discursive Limits of Sex*. New York: Routledge.

Campbell, F.A.K. (2008). Exploring Internalised Ableism Using Critical Race Theory. *Disability and Society, 23*(2), pp. 151–162.

Carey, N., Zlotowitz, S., James, S., Dennis, A., Gillspie, T., Hady, K. & The Housing & Mental Health Network. (2022). Building Alliances with Marginalised Communities to Challenge London's Unjust and Distressing Housing System. In Walker, C., Zoli, A. & Zlotowitz, S (eds.) *New Ideas for New Times: A Handbook of Innovative Community and Clinical Psychologies*. Switzerland: Palgrave.

Carlson, D.L., Wells, T.C., Mark, L. & Sandoval, J. (2021). Introduction: Working the Tensions of the Post-qualitative Movement in Qualitative Inquiry. *Qualitative Inquiry, 27*(2), pp. 151–157.

Chapman, R. (2019). Neurodiversity Theory and Its Discontents: Autism, Schizophrenia, and the Social Model of Disability. In Tekin, S. & Bluhm, R. (eds.) *The Bloomsbury Companion to Philosophy of Psychiatry*. New York: Bloomsbury Academic.

Charlton, J.I. (1998). *Nothing about Us without Us: Disability Oppression and Empowerment*. Berkeley: University of California Press.

Cheshmehzangi, A., Zou, T. & Su, Z. (2022). The Digital Divide Impacts on Mental Health during the COVID-19 Pandemic. *Brain, Behavior, and Immunity, 101*, pp. 211–213.

Chung, M.C. & Hyland, M.E. (2012). *History and Philosophy of Psychology*. London: Wiley Blackwell.

Coimbra, J.L., Duckett, P., Fryer, D., Makkawi, I., Menezes, I., Seedat, M. & Walker, C. (2012). Rethinking Community Psychology: Critical Insights. *The Australian Community Psychologist, 24*(2), pp. 135–142.

Collins, A.F. (1999). The Enduring Appeal of Physiognomy: Physical Appearance as a Sign of Temperament, Character, and Intelligence. *History of Psychology, 2*(4), pp. 251–276.

Condie, J. & Richards, M. (2022). *A Call for a Digital Community Psychology*. In Kagan, C., Akhurst, J., Alfaro, J., Lawthom, R., Richards, M. & Zambrano, A. (eds.) *The Routledge International Handbook of Community Psychology*. New York: Routledge.

Cordeiro, J. (2014). The Boundaries of the Human: From Humanism to Transhumanism. *World Futures Review, 6*(3), pp. 231–239.

Cordell, A. (1959). *Rape of the Fair Country*. London: Blorenge Books.

Craig, C.C. (2020). *Associationalism and the Literary Imagination: From the Phantasmal Chaos*. Scotland: Edinburgh University Press.

Dalton, J.H., Elias, M.J. & Wandersman, A. (Eds.). (2001). *Community Psychology: Linking Individuals and Communities*. London: Thomson Learning.

Davies, A.R., Honeyman, M. & Gann, B. (2021). Addressing the Digital Inverse Care Law in the Time of COVID-19: Potential for Digital Technology to Exacerbate or Mitigate Health Inequalities. *Journal of Medical Internet Research, 23*(4), pp. 4–22.

Deleuze, G. & Guattari, F. (1987). *A Thousand Plateaus: Capitalism and Schizophrenia.* London: Continuum.

Delio, I. (2012). Transhumanism or Ultrahumanism? Teilhard de Chardin on Technology, Religion and Evolution. *Theology and Science, 10*(2), pp. 153–166.

Derrida, J. (1997/2008). *The Animal That Therefore I Am.* New York: Fordham University Press.

Drake, E., Jeffrey, G. & Duckett, P. (2022). Colonised Minds and Community Psychology in the Academy: Collaborative Autoethnographic Reflections. *American Journal of Community Psychology, 69*(3–4), pp. 415–425.

Dutta, U. (2016). Prioritizing the Local in an Era of Globalization: A Proposal for Decentering Community Psychology. *American Journal of Community Psychology, 58*(3–4), pp. 329–338.

Dutta, U. (2018). Decolonising 'Community' in Community Psychology. *American Journal of Community Psychology, 62*(3–4), pp. 272–282.

Dzidic, P., Breen, L.J. & Bishop, B.J. (2013). Are Our Competencies Revealing Our Weaknesses? A Critique of Community Psychology Practice Competencies. *Global Journal of Community Psychology Practice, 4*(4), pp. 1–10.

Elkins, D.N. (2009). Why Humanistic Psychology Lost its Power and Influence in American Psychology. *Journal of Humanistic Psychology, 49*(3), pp. 267–291.

Evans, S.D., Duckett, P., Lawthom, R. & Kivell, N. (2017). *Positioning the Critical in Community Psychology.* In Bond, M.A., Serrano-García, I., Keys, C.B. & Shinn, M. (eds.) *APA Handbook of Community Psychology: Theoretical Foundations, Core Concepts, and Emerging Challenges* (pp. 107–127). Washington, DC: American Psychological Association.

Fanon, F. (1952/2008). *Black Skin, White Masks.* London: Penguin.

Fanon, F. (1967). *The Wretched of the Earth.* London: Penguin.

Ferrando, F. (2012). Towards A Posthumanist Methodology. A Statement. https://www.frameliteraryjournal.com/wp-content/uploads/2014/11/Frame-25_01-Ferrando.pdf

Ferrando, F. (2013). From the Eternal Recurrence to the Posthuman Multiverse'. In the Nietzsche Circle. *The Agonist, 4*(11), pp. 1–11.

Ferrando, F. (2014). The Posthuman' by Rosa Braidotti. In Ferrando, F. (ed.) *Plurilogue: Politics and Philosophy Review* (p. 229). New York: Polity.

Fisher, A.T., Sonn, C. & Evans, S.D. (2007). The Place and Function of Power in Community Psychology: Philosophical and Practical Issues. *Journal of Community & Applied Social Psychology, 17*, pp. 258–267.

Ford, D.H. & Urban, H.B. (1963). *Systems of Psychotherapy: A Comparative Study.* New York: John Wiley & Sons Inc.

Foucault, M. (1964). *Madness and Civilization: A History of Insanity in the Age of Reason.* New York: Vintage.

Foucault, M. (1972). *The Archaeology of Knowledge.* New York: Pantheon Books.

Foucault, M. (1977). *Discipline and Punish: The Birth of the Prison.* New York: Pantheon Books.

Foucault, M. (1978). *The History of Sexuality.* Volume 1: An Introduction. Pantheon Books: New York.

Fox, D., Prilleltensky, I. & Austin, S. (2009). Critical Psychology for Social Justice: Concerns and Dilemmas. In Fox, D., Prilleltensky, I. & Austin, S. (eds.) *Critical Psychology: An Introduction* (pp. 3–19). London: Sage Publications Ltd.

Fox, N.J. & Alldred, P. (2017). *Sociology and the New Materialism: Theory, Research, Action*. London: Sage.

Freire, P. (1970). *Pedagogy of the Oppressed*. London: Penguin.

Frigerio, A., Benozzo, A., Holmes, R. & Runswick-Cole, K. (2018). The Doing and Undoing of the 'Autistic Child': Cutting Together and apart Interview-Based Empirical Materials. *Qualitative Inquiry, 24*(6), p. 390.

Fritsch, K. (2010). Intimate Assemblages: Disability, Intercorporeality, and the Labour of Attendant Care. *Critical Disability Discourses, 2*. https://cdd.journals.yorku.ca/index.php/cdd/article/view/23854/28098.

Fromm, E. (1973). *The Anatomy of Human Destructiveness*. New York: Fawcett Crest.

Fryer, D. (2008). Some Questions about 'The History of Community Psychology'. *Journal of Community Psychology, 36*(5), pp. 572–586.

Fryer, D. & Fox, R. (2015). Community Psychology: Subjectivity, Power, Collectivity. In Parker, I. (ed.) *Handbook of Critical Psychology* (pp. 145–154). New York: Routledge.

Fryer, D. & Laing, A. (2008). Community Psychologies: What are They? What Could They Be? Why Does it Matter? A Critical Community Psychology Approach. *Australian Community Psychologist, 20*(2), pp. 7–15.

Gergen, K. (1973). Social Psychology as History. *Journal of Personality and Social Psychology, 26*, pp. 309–320.

Gibson, B.E. (2006). Disability, Connectivity and Transgressing the Autonomous Body. *Journal of Medical Humanities, 27*(3), pp. 187–196.

Gibson, B.E., Fadyl, J.K., Terry, G., Waterworth, K., Mosleh, D. & Kayes, N.M. (2021). A Posthuman Decentring of Person-Centred Care. *Health Sociology Review, 30*(3), pp. 292–307.

Gibson-Graham, J.K. (1999). Queer(y)ing Capitalism In and Out of the Classroom. *Journal of Geography in Higher Education, 23*(1), pp. 80–85.

Godfrey, M., Young, J. & Shannon, R. (2018). The Person, Interactions and Environment Programme to Improve Care of People with Dementia in Hospital: A Multisite Study. Southampton (UK): NIHR Journals Library; 2018 Jun. (Health Services and Delivery Research, No. 6.23.) Chapter 4, Person-centred Care: Meaning and Practice. Available from: https://www.ncbi.nlm.nih.gov/books/NBK508103/

Gomel, E. (2014). *Science Fiction, Alien Encounters and the Ethics of Posthumanism: Beyond the Golden Rule*. New York: Palgrave Macmillan.

Goodley, D. & Lawthom, R. (2005a). Epistemological Journeys in Participatory Action Research: Alliances between Community Psychology and Disability Studies. *Disability and Society, 20*(2), pp. 135–151.

Goodley, D. & Lawthom, R. (2005b). *Disability and Psychology: Critical Introductions and Reflections*. London: Palgrave.

Goodley, D. (2007). Becoming Rhizomatic Parents: Deleuze, Guattari and Disabled Babies. *Disability and Society, 22*(2), pp. 145–160.

Goodley, D. (2011). *Disability Studies: An Interdisciplinary Introduction*. London: Sage.

Goodley, D. (2013). Dis/entangling Critical Disability Studies. *Disability & Society, 28*(5), pp. 631–644.

Goodley, D. (2014). The Posthuman. *Disability and Society, 29*(5), pp. 844–846.

Goodley, D., Lawthom, R. & Runswick-Cole, K. (2014). Posthuman Disability Studies. *Subjectivity, 7*(4), p. 342.

Goodley, D. & Runswick-Cole, K. (2016). Becoming Dishuman: Thinking about the Human through Dis/Ability. *Discourse: Studies in the Cultural Politics of Education, 37*(1), pp. 1–15.

Goodley, D., Liddiard, K. & Runswick-Cole, K. (2017). Feeling Disability: Theories of Affect and Critical Disability Studies. *Disability and Society, 33*(2), pp. 197–217.

Goodley, D., Lawthom, R., Liddiard, K. & Runswick-Cole, K. (2019). Provocations for Critical Disability Studies. *Disability & Society, 34*(6), pp. 972–997.

Goodley, D. (2021). *Disability and Other Human Questions*. Bingley: Emerald Publishing Limited.

Goodley, D., Lawthom, R., Liddiard, L. & Runswick-Cole, K. (2022). Affect, Dis/ability and the Pandemic. *Sociology of Health and Illness,* https://onlinelibrary.wiley.com/doi/full/10.1111/1467-9566.13483.

Gough, B., McFadden, M. & McDonald, M. (2013). *Critical Social Psychology: An Introduction* (2nd ed.). London: Bloomsbury.

Gray, C.H. (2002). *Cyborg Citizen: Politics in the Posthuman Age*. London: Routledge.

Grech, S. (2009). Disability, Poverty, and Development: Critical Reflections on the Majority World Debate. *Disability and Society, 24*(6), pp. 771–784.

Grech, S. & Goodley, D. (2012). Doing Disability Research in the Majority World: An Alternative Framework and the Quest for Decolonising Methods. *Journal of Human Development, Disability and Social Change, 19*(2), pp. 43–55.

Grech, S. (2015). Decolonising Eurocentric Disability Studies: Why Colonialism Matters in the Disability and Global South Debate. *Social Identities, 21*(1), pp. 6–21.

Gridley H. & Breen L.J. (2007). So Far and Yet So Near? Community Psychology in Australia. In Reich, S.M., Riemer, M., Prilleltensky, I. & Montero, M. (eds.) *International Community Psychology* (pp. 119–139). Boston, MA: Springer.

Griffiths, M. (2022). Disabled Youth Participation within Activism and Social Movement Bases: An Empirical Investigation of the UK Disabled People's Movement. *Current Sociology,* https://journals.sagepub.com/doi/full/10.1177/00113921221100579.

Grünbaum, A. (1986). Précis of the Foundations of Psychoanalysis: A Philosophical Critique. *Behavioral and Brain Sciences, 9*(2), pp. 217–228.

Hadjiosif, M. & Desai, M. (2022). The Evolution of the Community Psychology Festival. In Walker, C., Zoli, A. & Zlotowitz, S (eds.) *New Ideas for New Times: A Handbook of Innovative Community and Clinical Psychologies*. Switzerland: Palgrave.

Halberstam, J. & Livingston, I. (1995). *Posthuman Bodies*. Bloomington: Indiana University Press.

Haraway, D. (1985/2006). A Cyborg Manifesto: Science, Technology, and Socialist-Feminism in the Late 20th Century. In Weiss, J., Nolan, J., Hunsinger, J. & Trifonas, P. (eds.) *The International Handbook of Virtual Learning Environments* (pp. 117–158). Dordrecht: Springer.

Haraway, D. (1991). *Simians, Cyborgs, and Women: The Reinvention of Nature*. New York: Routledge.

Harcourt, F. (2016). Wittgenstein and Psychoanalysis. In Glock, H.-J. & Hyman, J. (eds.) *A Companion to Wittgenstein*. Oxford: John Wiley and Sons.

Harré, R. & Second, P.F. (1972). *The Explanation of Social Behaviour*. Oxford: Blackwell.

Hassan, I. (1977). Prometheus as Performer: Toward a Posthumanist Culture? In Benamou, M. & Caramello, C. (eds.) *Performance in Postmodern Culture* (pp. 201–217) Madison, WI: Coda Press.

Hayles, N.K. (1999). *How We Became Posthuman*. Chicago, IL: Chicago University Press.

Henriksen, D., Creely, E. & Mehta, R. (2021). Rethinking the Politics of Creativity: Posthumanism, Indigeneity, and Creativity beyond the Western Anthropocene. *Qualitative Inquiry, 28*(5), pp. 465–475.

Herbrechter, S. (2013). *Posthumanism and Science Fiction: A Critical Analysis*. London: Bloomsbury Academic.

Herbrechter, S. (2017). Posthumanism and Educational Research. *Educational Philosophy and Theory, 49*(11), pp. 1125–1127.

Hoffman, L., Cleare-Hoffman, H., Granger, N. & St John, D. (2020). *To Multiculturalism and Diversity: Perspectives on Existence and Difference*. New York: Routledge.

Holdstock, L. (1993). *Can We Afford not to Revision the Person-centred Concept of Self?* In Brazier, D. (ed.) *Beyond Carl Rogers* (pp. 229–252). London: Constable.

Holman-Jones, S. (2016). Living Bodies of Thought: The Critical in Critical Autoethnography. *Qualitative Inquiry, 22*(2), pp. 228–237.

Hughes, J. (2004). *Citizen Cyborg: Why Democratic Societies Must Respond to the Redesigned Human of the Future*. Cambridge, MA: Westview Press.

Hughes, B. & Paterson, K. (2006). The Social Model of Disability and the Disappearing Body: Towards a Sociology of Impairment. In Barton, L. (ed.) *Overcoming Disabling Barriers: 18 Years of Disability and Society* (pp. 27–35). London: Routledge.

Hughes, B. (2009). Wounded/Monstrous/Abject: A Critique of the Disabled Body in the Sociological Imaginary. *Disability & Society, 24*(4), pp. 399–410.

Hughes, B. (2012). Fear, Pity and Disgust: Emotions and the Non-Disabled Imaginary. In Watson, N., Roulstone, A. & Thomas, C. (eds.) *Routledge Handbook of Disability Studies* (pp. 67–78). London: Routledge.

Hughes, B.M. (2018). *Psychology in Crisis*. London: Palgrave.

Hyland, M. (2020). *A History of Psychology in Ten Questions*. New York: Routledge.

Israel, J. & Tajfel, H. (eds.) (1972). *The Context of Social Psychology: A Critical Assessment*. London: Academic Press.

Kagan, C., Duggan, K., Richards, M. & Siddiquee, A. (2011). Community Psychology. In Martin, P., Cheung, F., Kyrios, M., Littlefield, L., Knowles, M., Overmier, B. & Prieto, J.M. (eds.) *The IAAP Handbook of Applied Psychology* (pp. 471–500). Oxford: Blackwell.

Kagan, C., Burton, M., Duckett, P., Lawthom, R. & Siddiquee, A. (2021). *Critical Community Psychology: Critical Action and Social Change*. London: Routledge.

Kagan, C., Akhurst, J., Alfaro, J., Lawthom, R., Richards, M. & Zambrano, A. (2022). *The Routledge International Handbook of Community Psychology*. New York: Routledge.

Kaiser, M.S., Al Mamun, S., Mahmud, M. & Tania, M.H. (2021). Healthcare Robots to Combat COVID-19. In Santosh, K. & Joshi, A. (eds.) *COVID-19: Prediction, Decision-Making, and its Impacts. Lecture Notes on Data Engineering and Communications Technologies*, vol. 60. Singapore: Springer.

Kaufman, A.S. (1999). Intelligence Tests and School Psychology: Predicting the Future by Studying the Past. *Psychology of Schools, 37*(1), pp. 7–16.

Kelly, J.G. (1968). Toward an Ecological Conception of Preventive Interventions. In Carter, J.S. (ed.), *Research Contributions from Psychology to Community Mental Health* (pp. 75–99). New York: Behavioral Publications.

Kerr, J. (1968). *The Tiger Who Came to Tea*. London: Collins.

Kessi, S., Suffla, S. & Seedat, M. (2021). Towards A Decolonial Community Psychology: Derivatives, Disruptions and Disobediences. Springer. In Kessi, S., Suffla, S. & Seedat, M. (eds.) *Decolonial Enactments in Community Psychology. Community Psychology.* Springer.

King, D.B., Woody, W.D. & Viney, W. (2013). *A History of Psychology: Ideas and Context.* New York: Routledge.

Kloos, B., Hill, J., Thomas, E., Case, A.D., Scott, V.C. & Wandersman, A. (2021). *Community Psychology: Linking Individuals and Communities* (4th ed.). Washington, DC: American Psychological Association.

Kumm, B.E., Berbary, L.A. & Grimwood, B.S.R. (2019). For Those to Come: An Introduction to Why Posthumanism Matters. *Leisure Sciences, 41*(5), pp. 341–347.

Laing, R.D. (1965). *The Divided Self: An Existential Study in Sanity and Madness.* Harmondsworth: Penguin.

Laing, R.D. (1969). *Self and Others.* (2nd ed.). London: Penguin Books.

Lawthom, R., Kagan, C. & Sixsmith, J. (2007). Interrogating Power: The Case of Arts and Mental Health in Community Projects. *Journal of Community Applied Social Psychology, 17*(4), pp. 268–279.

Lawthom, R., Kagan, C., Richards, M., Sixsmith, J. & Woolrych, R. (2012) Being Creative: Engaging and Participative Methodologies. In Johnson, S. & Horrocks, C. (eds.) *Advances in Health Psychology: Critical Approaches* (pp. 204–220). Basingstoke: Palgrave.

Leahey, T.H. (1992). The Mythical Revolutions of American Psychology. *American Psychologist, 47*(2), pp. 308–318.

Leplege, A., Gzil, F., Cammelli, M., Lefeve, C., Pachoud, B. & Ville, I. (2007). Person-Centredness: Conceptual and Historical Perspectives. *Disability and Rehabilitation, 29*(20–21), pp. 1555–1565.

Levinas, E. (1977/1995). *Totalidad e infinito (Ensayo sobre la exterioridad). [Totality and infinity. An essay on exteriority].* Salamanca: Sígueme.

Liddiard, K. (2014). The Work of Disabled Identities in Intimate Relationships. *Disability and Society, 29*(1), pp. 115–128.

Liddiard, K., Whitney, S., Evans, K., Watts, L., Vogelmann, E., Spurr, R., Aimes, C., Runswick-Cole, K. & Goodley, D. (2019). Working the Edges of Posthuman Disability Studies: Theorising with Disabled Young People with Life-limiting Impairments. *Sociology of Health and Illness, 41*(8), pp. 1473–1487.

Liddiard, K. (2020). Surviving Ableism in Covid Times. https://kirstyliddiard.wordpress.com/2020/06/16/surviving-ableism-in-covid-times-only-the-vulnerable-will-be-at-risk-but-your-only-is-my-everything/

Logue, A. (1985). The Origins of Behaviorism: Antecedents and Proclamation. In Buxton, C.E. (ed.) *Points of View in the Modern History of Psychology.* Orlando, FL: Academic Press.

Lykes, M.B. & Moane, G. (2009). Whither Feminist Liberation Psychology? Critical Explorations of Feminist and Liberation Psychologies for a Globalizing World. *Feminism and Psychology, 19*(3), pp. 283–297.

Lyotard, J.F. (1979/1984). *The Postmodern Condition: A Report on Knowledge.* Minneapolis, MN: University of Minneapolis Press.

Maldonando-Torres, N. (2017). Frantz Fanon and the Decolonial Turn in Psychology: From Modern/Colonial Methods to the Decolonial Attitude. *South African Journal of Psychology, 47*(4), pp. 432–441.

Malherbe, N., Suffla, S. & Seedat, M. (2022). Epistemicide and Epistemic Freedom: Reflections for a Decolonising Community Psychology. In Kagan, C.,

Akhurst, J., Alfaro, J., Lawthom, R., Richards, M. & Zambrano, A. (eds.) *The Routledge International Handbook of Community Psychology.* New York: Routledge.

Manalastas, E.J., Muyargas, M.M., Docena, P.S. & Torre, B.A. (2022). Psychologists Taking Action for LGBT+ rights and Well-being in the Philippines. In Kagan, C., Akhurst, J., Alfaro, J., Lawthom, R., Richards, M. & Zambrano, A. (eds.) *The Routledge International Handbook of Community Psychology.* New York: Routledge.

Martin-Baro, I. (1994). *Writings for a Liberation Psychology.* Cambridge, MA: Harvard University Press.

Masson, J. (1988). *Against Therapy.* London: Fontana/Collins.

Massumi, B. (1992). *A User's Guide to Capitalism and Schizophrenia: Deviations from Deleuze and Guattari.* Cambridge, MA: MIT Press.

May, R. (1969). *Love and Will.* New York: Norton.

Meekosha, H. & Shuttleworth, R. (2009). What's so critical about critical disability studies? *Australian Journal of Human Rights, 15*(1), pp. 47–76.

Mehl, P.J. (2010). *Thinking through Kierkegaard: Existential Identity in a Pluralistic World.* Champaign: University of Illinois Press.

Miah, A. (2007). Posthumanism: A Critical History. In Gordijn, B. & Chadwick, R. (eds.) *Medical Enhancements & Posthumanity.* New York: Routledge.

Mignolo, W. & Walsh, C. (2018). *On Decoloniality: Concepts, Analytics, Praxis.* Durham, NC & London: Duke University Press.

Miles-Novelo, A. & Anderson, C.A. (2019). Climate Change and Psychology: Effects of Rapid Global Warming on Violence and Aggression. *Current Climate Change Reports, 5*, pp. 36–46.

Miller, G. (1969). Psychology as a Means of Promoting Human Welfare. *American Psychologist, 24*, pp. 1063–1075.

Montero, M. (2012). From Complexity and Social Justice to Consciousness: Ideas that Have Built a Community Psychology. *Global Journal of Community Psychology Practice, 3*(1), pp. 1–13.

Montero, M., Sonn, C.C. & Burton, M. (2017). Community Psychology and Liberation Psychology: A Creative Synergy for an Ethical and Transformative Praxis. In Bond, M.A., Serrano-García, I., Keys, C.B. & Shinn, M. (eds.) *APA Handbook of Community Psychology: Theoretical Foundations, Core Concepts, and Emerging Challenges* (pp. 149–167). American Psychological Association.

Morris, J. (2018). *Wonderings and Wanderings.* London: Page Publishing.

Murphy, D. & Joseph, S. (2019). Contributions from the Person-Centred Experiential Approach to the Field of Social Pedagogy. *Cambridge Journal of Education, 49*(2), pp. 181–196.

Murray, H. (2014). "My Place Was Set At The Terrible Feast": The Meanings of the "Anti-Psychiatry" Movement and Responses in the United States, 1970s–1990s. *The Journal of American Culture, 37*(1), pp. 37–51.

Naldemiric, O., Lydahl, D., Britten, N., Elam, M., Moore, L. & Wolf, A. (2016). Tenacious Assumptions of Person-Centred Care? Exploring Tensions and Variations in Practice. *Health: An Interdisciplinary Journal for the Social Study of Health, Illness and Medicine, 22*(1), pp. 54–71.

Nayar, P.K. (2014). *Posthumanism.* Cambridge: Wiley.

Nelson, G. & Prilleltensky, I. (2005). *Community Psychology: In Pursuit of Liberation and Well-Being.* New York: Palgrave Macmillan.

O'Donnell, R.P. (2011). Posthuman: Exploring the Obsolescence of the Corporeal Body in Contemporary Art. *Student Pulse the International Student Journal, 3*(8), p. 1.

O'Hara, M. (2015). *Austerity Bites: A Journey to the Sharp End of Cuts in the UK*. Bristol: Policy Press.

Office of National Statistics (2021). Outcomes for Disabled People in the UK, 2021. https://www.ons.gov.uk/peoplepopulationandcommunity/healthandsocialcare/disability/articles/outcomesfordisabledpeopleintheuk/2021

Oliver, M. (1990). *The Politics of Disablement*. Basingstoke: Macmillan and St Martin's Press.

Pailhez, G. & Bulbena, A. (2010). Body Shape and Psychiatric Diagnosis Revisited. *International Journal of Psychiatry in Clinical Practice, 14*(4), pp. 236–243.

Palmer, K.M. (2016[2018]). Psychology is in Crisis Over Whether it is a Crisis. In Hughes (ed.) *Psychology in Crisis*. London: Palgrave.

Parker, I. (2007). *Revolution in Psychology: Alienation to Emancipation*. London: Pluto.

Parker, I. (2020). *Psychology through Critical Autoethnography*. London: Routledge.

Parker, I. (2022). *Radical Psychoanalysis and Anti-Capitalist Action*. London: Resistance Books.

Popper, K. (2002). *The Logic of Scientific Discovery* (J.F.K. Popper & L. Freed, Trans.). New York: Routledge Classics.

Poulos, C.N. (2006). The Ties that Bind Us, the Shadows that Separate Us: Life and Death, Shadow and (dream)story. *Qualitative Inquiry, 12*, pp. 96–117.

Prilleltensky, I. (2019). Mattering at the Intersection of Psychology, Philosophy and Politics. *American Journal of Community Psychology, 65*(1–2), pp. 16–34.

Proctor, G., Cooper, M., Sanders, P. & Malcolm, B. (2006). *Politicising the Person-Centred Approach: An Agenda for Social Change*. Ross-on-Wye: PCCS Books.

Quayle, A.F. & Sonn, C.C. (2019). Amplifying the Voices of Indigenous Elders through Community Arts and Narrative Inquiry: Stories of Oppression, Psychosocial Suffering, and Survival. *American Journal of Community Psychology, 64*(1–2), pp. 46–58.

Rappaport, J. (1977). *Community Psychology: Values, Research and Action*. New York: Holt, Rinehart and Winston.

Reason, P. (1994). *Participation in Human Inquiry*. London: SAGE.

Reason, P. & Bradbury, H. (2001). Introduction: Inquiry and Participation in Search of a World Worthy of Human Aspiration. In Reason, P. & Bradbury, H. (eds.) *Handbook of Action Research: Participative Inquiry and Practice* (pp. 1–14). London: SAGE.

Reavey, P. (2021). *A Handbook of Visual Methods in Psychology: Using and Interpreting Images in Psychology*. New York: Routledge.

Reich, S.M. & Reich, J.A. (2006). Cultural Competence in Interdisciplinary Collaborations: A Method for Respecting Diversity in Research Partnerships. *American Journal of Community Psychology, 36*, pp. 51–62.

Reich, S.M., Riemer, M., Prilleltensky, I. & Montero, M. (2007). *International Community Psychology – History and Theories*. New York: Springer.

Research Excellence Framework (2021). Overview Report by Main Panel A and Sub-Panels 1–6, 2022.

Richards, M. (2014a). *Confessions of a Community Psychology: The Tale of a Group of Men Challenging the Perceptions of Health Promotion and Learning Difficulties* (Unpublished PhD thesis). Manchester Metropolitan University, Manchester.

Richards, M. (2014b). Reflecting on Identity and Context: Rapping Poetry with Marginalised Young Men. https://michaelrichards1983.wordpress.com/2014/

09/26/reflecting-on-identity-and-context-rapping-poetry-with-marginalised-young-men/

Richards, M. (2015a). Turning Back to the Story of My Life: An Autoethnographic Exploration of a Researcher's Identity during the PhD Process. *Journal of Reflective Practice: International and Multidisciplinary Perspectives, 16*(6), pp. 821–835.

Richards, M. (2015b). Book Review: 'Posthumanism' (2014) by Pramod K. Nayar. https://michaelrichards1983.wordpress.com/2015/08/19/book-review-posthumanism-2014-by-pramod-k-nayer/

Richards, M. (2016a). People with Learning Disabilities Need a Commissioner and a Legal Charter of Rights'–No They Do Not! *Disability & Society, 31*(3), pp. 426–430.

Richards, M. (2016b). 'You've got autism because you like order and you do not look into my eyes': Some Reflections on Understanding the Label of 'Autism Spectrum Disorder' from a Dishuman Perspective. *Disability and Society, 31*(9), pp. 1–5.

Richards, M. (2017). 'Angry, when things don't go my own way': What It Means to be Gay with Learning Disabilities. *Disability & Society, 32*(8), pp. 1165–1179.

Richards, M., Lawthom, R. & Runswick-Cole, K. (2018). Community-based Arts Research for People with Learning Disabilities: Challenging Misconceptions about Learning Disabilities. *Disability and Society, 34*(2), pp. 204–227.

Richards, M. (2019). Whorlton Hall, Winterbourne … Person-centred Care is Long Dead for People with Learning Disabilities and Autism. *Disability & Society, 35*(3), pp. 500–505.

Richards, M. (2022). 'I am not disabled, I just need some help': Are Critical Community Psychology Approaches a Promising Way to Engage with People with Learning Disabilities? In Walker, C., Zoli, A. & Zlotowitz, S (eds.) *New Ideas for New Times: A Handbook of Innovative Community and Clinical Psychologies.* Switzerland: Palgrave.

Richardson, L. & St. Pierre, E.A. (2005). Writing: A Method of Inquiry. In Denzin, N. & Lincoln, Y. (eds.) *Handbook of Qualitative Research* (pp. 959–978). Thousand Oaks, CA: Sage.

Richert, L. (2019). *Break on Through: Radical Psychiatry and the American Counterculture.* Cambridge: The MIT Press.

Rickel, A.U. (1987). The 1965 Swampscott Conference and Future Topics for Community Psychology. *American Journal of Community Psychology, 15*(5), pp. 511–513.

Rock, M.J., Degeling, C. & Blue, G. (2014). Towards Stronger Theory in Critical Public Health: Insights from Debates Surrounding Posthumanism. *Critical Public Health, 24*(3), pp. 337–348.

Roets, G. & Goedgeluck, M. (2007). Daisies on the Road. *Qualitative Inquiry, 13*(1), pp. 85–112.

Roets, G. & Goodley, D. (2008). Citizenship and Uncivilised Society: The Smooth and Nomadic Qualities of Self-advocacy. *Disability Studies Quarterly, 28*(4), pp. 1–8.

Rogers, C.R. (1980/1995). *A Way of Being.* Boston: Houghton Mifflin Company.

Rosenthal, L. (2016). Incorporating Intersectionality into Psychology: An Opportunity to Promote Social Justice and Equity. *American Psychologist, 71*(6), pp. 474–485.

Saher, R. & Anjum, M. (2021). Role of Technology in COVID-19 Pandemic. History, Diagnostic Tools, Epidemiology, Healthcare and Technology. In Hameed, K., Bhatia, S., Ahmed, S.T., Bhattacharyya, S. & Dey, N. (eds.) *Researches and Applications of Artificial Intelligence to Mitigate Pandemics* (pp. 109–138). Academic Press.

Saltzman, L.Y., Hansel, T.C. & Bordnick, P.S. (2020). Loneliness, Isolation, and Social Support Factors in Post-COVID-19 Mental Health. *Psychological Trauma: Theory, Research, Practice, and Policy, 12*(S1), pp. S55–S57.

Sanders, P. (2017). *Principled and Strategic Opposition to the Medicalisation of Distress and all of its Apparatus.* In Joseph, S. (ed.) *Person-Centred Therapy and Mental Health* (2nd ed.). Ross-on-Wye: PCCS Books.

Schumacher, L. (2011). *Divine Illumination – The History and Future of Augustine's Theory of Knowledge.* Chichester: John Wiley and Sons Ltd.

Scott-Samuel, A., Bambra, C., Collins, C., Hunter, D.J., McCartney, G. & Smith, K. (2014). The Impact of Thatcherism on Health and Well-Being in Britain. *International Journal of Health Services, 44*(1), pp. 53–71.

Shakespeare, T. & Corker, M. (2002). *Disability/Postmodernity: Embodying Disability Theory.* London: Continuum.

Shakespeare, T. & Watson, N. (2002). The Social Model of Disability: An Outdated Ideology? *Research in Social Science and Disability, 2,* pp. 9–28.

Shildrick, M. (2007). Contested Pleasures: The Sociopolitical Economy of Disability and Sexuality. *Sexuality Research and Social Policy, 4*(1), pp. 53–66.

Shildrick, M. (2009). *Dangerous Discourses of Disability, Subjectivity and Sexuality.* Basingstoke: Palgrave Macmillan.

Simpson, P. & Richards, M. (2018). Using Photovoice with Working-class Men: Affordances, Contradictions, and Limits to Reflexivity. *Qualitative Research in Psychology, 19*(1), pp. 155–175.

Slater, J. (2015). *Youth and Disability: A Challenge to Mr Reasonable.* Abingdon: Ashgate Publishing.

Sloan, T. (1996). *Damaged Life: The Crisis of the Modern Psyche.* New York: Routledge.

Smail, D. (1994). Community Psychology and Politics. *Journal of Community and Applied Social Psychology, 4*(1), pp. 3–10.

Sonn, C.C. (2016). Swampscott in International Context: Expanding Our Ecology of Knowledge. *American Journal of Community Psychology, 58*(3–4), pp. 309–313.

Sonn, C.C., Fox, R., Keast, S. & Rua, M. (2022a). Fostering and Sustaining Transnational Solidarities for Transformative Social Change: Advancing Community Psychology Research and Action. *American Journal of Community Psychology, 69*(3–4), pp. 269–282.

Sonn, C.C., Quayle, A.F. & Balla, P. (2022b). Community Arts for Critical Community Psychology Praxis: Towards Decolonialisation and Aboriginal Self-Determination. In Kagan, C., Akhurst, J., Alfaro, J., Lawthom, R., Richards, M. & Zambrano, A. (2022). *The Routledge International Handbook of Community Psychology.* New York: Routledge.

Springborg, P. (2016). Hobbes's Materialism and Epicurean Mechanism. *British Journal for the History of Philosophy, 24*(5), pp. 814–835.

Stein, C.H., Hartl-Majcher, J., Froemming, M.W., Greenberg, S.C., Benoit, M.F., Gonzales, S.M., Petrowski, C.E., Mattei, G.M. & Dulek, E.B. (2019). Community Psychology, Digital Technology, and Loss: Remembrance Activities of Young Adults Who Have Experienced the Death of a Close Friend. *Journal of Community and Applied Social Psychology, 29*(4), pp. 257–272.

Stephens, E. & Cryle, P. (2017). Eugenics and the Normal Body: The Role of Visual Images and Intelligence Testing in Framing the Treatment of People with Disabilities in the Early Twentieth Century. *Continuum, 31*(3), pp. 365–376.

Stevens, G. & Sonn, C.C. (2021). *Decoloniality and Epistemic Justice in Contemporary Community Psychology*. Cham: Springer.

Strudwick, G., Sockalingam, S., Kassam, I., Sequiera, L., Bonato, S., Youssef, A., Mehta, R., Green., N., Agic, B., Soklaridis, S., Impey, D., Wilier, D. & Crawford, A. (2021). Digital Interventions to Support Population Mental Health in Canada during the COVID-19 Pandemic: Rapid Review. *JMIR Mental Health, 8*(3), https://scholar.google.com/citations?view_op=view_citation&hl=en&user=5-V3UikAAAAJ&citation_for_view=5-V3UikAAAAJ:aqlVkmm33-oC.

Szasz, T. (1961). *The Myth of Mental Illness*. New York: Penguin.

Tebes, J.K. (2016). Reflections on the Future of Community Psychology from the Generations after Swampscott: A Commentary and Introduction to the Special Issue. *American Journal of Community Psychology*, 58, pp. 229–238.

Tironi, E., Barrett, D., Rayner, D., Dillane, S., Trapolini, T., Hewitt, R., Henry, E. & Rhodes, P. (2022). World Eco-Psychology: A Collective Bio-Ethnography. *Arena of Ecology*, https://link.springer.com/article/10.1007/s42087-022-00274-x.

Toro, J. & Martiny, K. (2020). New Perspectives on Person-Centred Care: An Affordance-Based Account. *Medicine, Health Care and Philosophy, 23*, pp. 631–644.

Tremain, S. (2005). Foucault, Governmentality, and Critical Disability Theory. In Tremain, S. (ed.) *Foucault and the Government of Disability* (pp. 1–25). Michigan: University of Michigan Press.

Trickett, E.J. (2009). Community Psychology: Individuals and Interventions in Community Context. *Annual Review of Psychology, 60*, pp. 395–419.

Trott, C.D., Reimer-Watts, K. & Reimer, M. (2022). Climate Justice: In Pursuit of a Practical Utopia: Transitioning Towards Climate Justice. In Kagan, C., Akhurst, J., Alfaro, J., Lawthom, R., Richards, M. & Zambrano, A. (2022). *The Routledge International Handbook of Community Psychology*. New York: Routledge.

Tudor, K. (2016). Critiques of Person-Centred Theory – From Within and From Outside the Person-Centred Nation. In Lago, C. & Charura, D. (eds.) *The Person-Centred Counselling and Psychotherapy Handbook: Origins, Developments and Current Applications*. Berkshire: Open University Press.

Tudor, K. & Worrall, M. (2006). *Person-Centred Therapy: A Clinical Philosophy*. New York: Routledge.

Ulmer, J.B. (2017). Posthumanism as Research Methodology: Inquiry in the Anthropocene. *International Journal of Qualitative Studies in Education*, 30(9), pp. 832–848.

Van Belle, H. (1980). *Basic Intent and Therapeutic Approach of Carl R. Rogers*. Toronto: Wedge.

Vazquez Rivera, C. (2010). *International Community Psychology. Shared Agendas in Diversity*. San Juan: CIREC, University of Porto Rico.

Vehmas, S. & Watson, N. (2013). Moral Wrongs, Disadvantages, and Disability: A Critique of Critical Disability Studies. *Disability and Society, 29*(4), pp. 638–650.

Vint, S. (2022). The Biopolitics of Posthumanism in Tears in Rain. In Daigle, C. & McDonald, T.H. (eds.) *Deleuze and Guattari to Posthumanism – Philosophies of Immanence*. London: Bloomsbury.

Vitz, P.C. (1977[1994]). *Psychology as Religion: The Cult of Self-worship* (2nd ed.). Grand Rapids, MI: Eerdmans.

Walker, C., Zoli, A. & Zlotowitz, S. (2022) (eds.) *New Ideas for New Times: A Handbook of Innovative Community and Clinical Psychologies*. New York: Palgrave.

Wassmann, C. (2010). Reflections on the "Body Loop": CARL Georg Lange's Theory of Emotion. *Cognition and Emotion, 24*(6), pp. 974–990.

Watermeyer, B. & Swartz, L. (2008). Conceptualising the Psycho-emotional Aspects of Disability and Impairment: The Distortion of Personal and Psychic Boundaries. *Disability in Society, 23*(6), pp. 599–610.

Watermeyer, B. (2012). Is it Possible to Create a Politically Engaged, Contextual Psychology of Disability? *Disability and Society, 27*(2), pp. 161–174.

Watermeyer, B. (2019). "Can This White Guy Sing the Blues?" Disability, Race, and Decolonisation in South African Higher Education. In Watermeyer, B., McKenzie, J. & Swartz, L. (eds.) *The Palgrave Handbook of Disability and Citizenship in the Global South*. New York: Palgrave Macmillan.

Watkins, M. (2015). Psychsocial Accompaniment. *Journal of Social and Political Psychology, 3*(1), pp. 324–341.

Watkins, M. (2021). Toward a Decolonial Approach to Psychosocial Accompaniment from the "Outside". In Stevens, G. & Sonn, C.C. (eds.) *Decoloniality and Epistemic Justice in Contemporary Community Psychology. Community Psychology*. New York: Springer.

Watson, J.B. (19131948). Psychology as the Behaviorist Views It, 1913. In Dennis, W. (ed.) *Readings in the History of Psychology* (pp. 457–471). New York: Appleton.

Wenger, E. (1998). *Communities of Practice: Learning, Meaning, and Identity*. Cambridge, MA: Cambridge University Press.

Whitehead, P.M. (2018). *Expanding the Category 'Human': Nonhumanism, Posthumanism and Humanistic Psychology*. London: Lexington Books.

Willig, C. (2015). *Discourse Analysis*. In Smith, J.A. (ed.) *Qualitative Psychology: A Practical Guide to Research Methods*. Sage.

Wilson, S. (2006). *Corpus' from Sensorium – Embodied Experience, Technology, and Contemporary Art*. Cambridge, MA: MIT Press.

Winfield, A.G. (2012). Resuscitating Bad Science: Eugenics Past and Present. In Watkins, W.H. (ed.) *The Assault on Public Education*. New York: Teachers College Press.

Wolfe, C. (2010). *What is Posthumanism?* Minnesota: University of Minnesota Press.

Young, S. (2006). *Designer Evolution – A Transhumanist Manifesto*. New York: Prometheus Books.

Zoli, A., Ackhurst, J., Di Martino, S. & Bochicchio, D. (2022). Overcoming Marginalisation and Mental Distress Through Community Supported Agriculture: The Streccapogn Experience in Monteveglio, Italy. In Walker, C., Zoli, A. & Zlotowitz, S (eds.) *New Ideas for New Times: A Handbook of Innovative Community and Clinical Psychologies*. New York: Palgrave.

Index

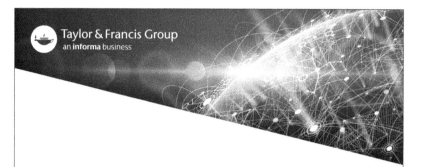